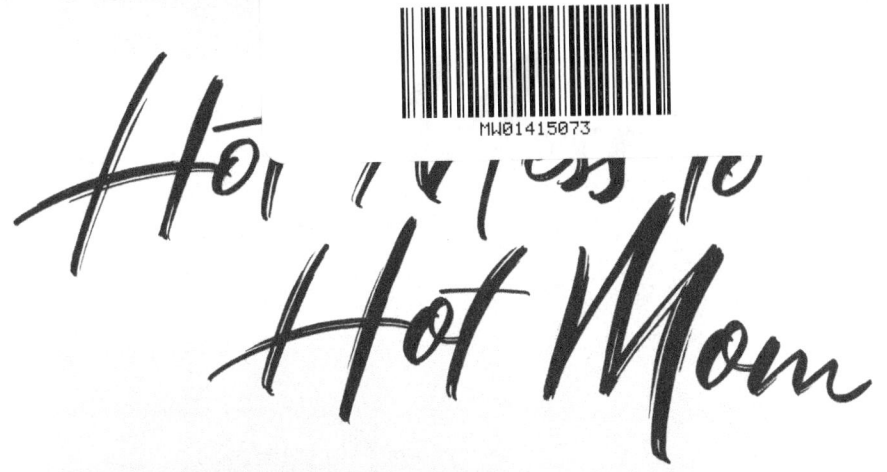

Hot Mess to Hot Mom

TRANSFORMATIONAL TOOLS FOR THRIVING AFTER CHILDBIRTH AND BEYOND

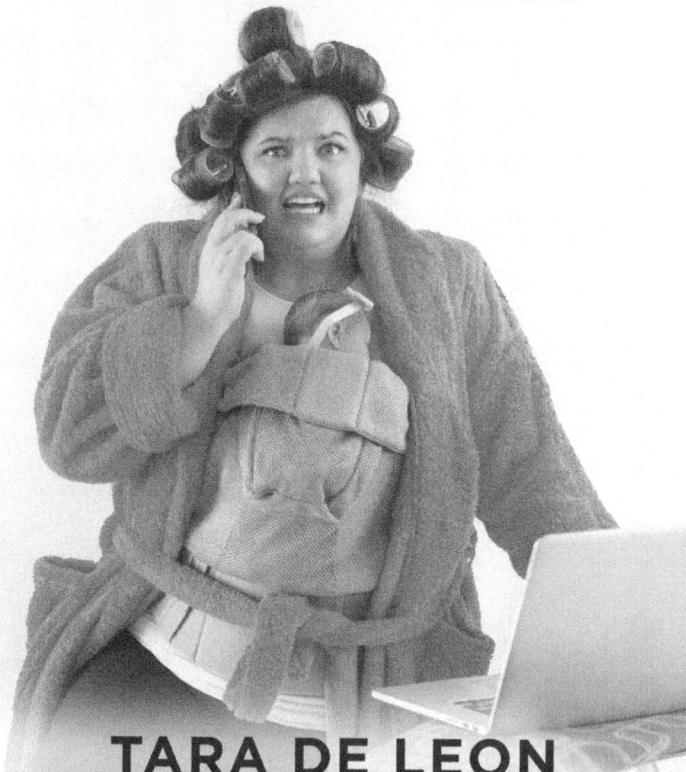

TARA DE LEON

FEATURING: VALERIE E. ANIAS, ROBIN LEE ARNESEN, JULIE BLAMPHIN, TRISH BREWER, BETH CONLON, AUBREY EDWARDS, DR. GINA HAHN, ELIZABETH HARRIS, ALICEANNE LOFTUS, KAITLYN MARTIN, MELISSA MAXWELL, KELLY MYERSON, TOMIKA ROBERTSON, SHELLY SCHOFF, MELISSA SZUROVY, DR. IRUM TAHIR, MARIA WINTERS

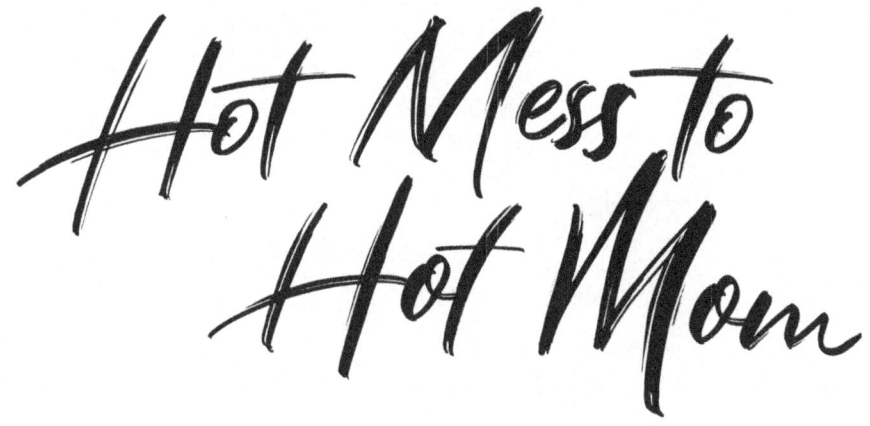

TRANSFORMATIONAL TOOLS FOR THRIVING
AFTER CHILDBIRTH AND BEYOND

TARA DE LEON

FEATURING: VALERIE E. ANIAS, ROBIN LEE ARNESEN, JULIE BLAMPHIN,
TRISH BREWER, BETH CONLON, AUBREY EDWARDS, DR. GINA HAHN,
ELIZABETH HARRIS, ALICEANNE LOFTUS, KAITLYN MARTIN,
MELISSA MAXWELL, KELLY MYERSON, TOMIKA ROBERTSON,
SHELLY SCHOFF, MELISSA SZUROVY, DR. IRUM TAHIR, MARIA WINTERS

Tara De Leon

Copyright © 2024 Tara De Leon

Published by Brave Healer Productions

All rights reserved. No part of this book may be used or reproduced by any means, graphic, electronic, or mechanical, including photocopying, recording, taping, or by any information storage retrieval system without the written permission of the publisher, except in the case of brief quotations embodied in critical articles and reviews.

Cover photograph © Maureen Porto Studios

Paperback ISBN: 978-1-961493-25-4

eBook ISBN: 978-1-961493-24-7

Dedication

To all the hot mess mamas out there. You are seen, heard, and loved. Now go act like the hot mom that you are.

And to my son, who made me a hot mom. Mavs, I love you, baby dude!

DISCLAIMER

This book offers health and nutritional information and is designed for educational purposes only. You should not rely on this information as a substitute for, nor does it replace professional medical advice, diagnosis, or treatment. If you have any concerns or questions about your health, you should always consult with a physician or other healthcare professional. Do not disregard, avoid, or delay obtaining medical or health-related advice from your healthcare professional because of something you may have read here. The use of any information provided in this book is solely at your own risk.

Any legal information provided in this book does not and is not intended to constitute legal advice or create an attorney client relationship; instead, all information, content and references are for general informational purposes only. Readers should contact an attorney directly to obtain advice with respect to any particular legal matter.

Developments in medical research may impact the health, fitness, and nutritional advice that appears here. No assurances can be given that the information contained in this book will always include the most relevant findings or developments with respect to the particular material.

Having said all that, know that the experts here have shared their tools, practices, and knowledge with you with a sincere and generous intent to assist you on your health and wellness journey. Please contact them with any questions you may have about the techniques or information they provided. They will be happy to assist you further!

Table of Contents

INTRODUCTION | i

Chapter 1
REBUILDING STRENGTH | 1
GENTLE EXERCISES FOR POSTPARTUM RECOVERY
By Tara De Leon, MS, RSCC, CSCS*D, Speaker, Mama

Chapter 2
RESTLESS TO RESTFUL | 16
SIMPLE STEPS FOR MOMS TO GET GREAT SLEEP
By Kelly Myerson, MA, OTR

Chapter 3
RUNNING STRONG:
NAVIGATING YOUR MOTHER RUNNER PACE | 25
AN EMPOWERED APPROACH TO SAFELY RUN POSTPARTUM
By Melissa Szurovy, RRCA Certified Run Coach

Chapter 4
42 DAYS FOR 42 YEARS | 38
SIMPLE POSTPARTUM RITUALS FOR LIFELONG HEALTH

By Melissa Maxwell, Ayurveda Health Counselor, RYT-500

Chapter 5
WHAT TO DO WHEN
THE CAT IN THE HAT IS YOU | 49
FOLLOWING YOUR FUN INTO A LIFE YOU LOVE

By Robin Lee Arnesen, Pilates Teacher

Chapter 6
THE MYTH OF THE GOOD MOTHER | 58
HOW TO ASK FOR HELP

By Maria Winters, LCPC, NCC

Chapter 7
THINK OUTSIDE THE BOX | 68
FIVE CREATIVE WAYS TO GET YOUR SEXY BACK

By Julie Blamphin, Speaker, Founder of Stretch Your Spirit

Chapter 8
MARRIAGE, BABY, AND BUSINESS, OH MY! | 79
NAVIGATING A GOOD OPPORTUNITY
WITH SEEMINGLY BAD TIMING.

By AliceAnne Loftus, Entrepreneur, Business and Leadership Coach

Chapter 9
YOUR BODY HAS CHANGED | 88
HONOR IT WITH CURIOSITY AND REST
By Dr. Gina Hahn, DPT, RKC

Chapter 10
MOTHERHOOD IS HARD. EATING DOESN'T HAVE TO BE. | 97
HEALTHY EATING SIMPLIFIED
By Elizabeth Harris, MS, RDN, Certified Intuitive Eating Counselor

---

Chapter 11
CULTIVATING A VILLAGE | 107
THE SUPPORT PARENTS WANT, BUT CHILDREN NEED
By Tomika Robertson

Chapter 12
A POSITIVE SPIN ON PARENTING | 116
HOW TO KEEP THE VIBE HIGH EVEN IN YOUR FRUSTRATING MOMENTS
By Aubrey Edwards, CEO, Bright Beginning Children's Learning Center

---

Chapter 13
HOW TO CALM YOUR NERVOUS SYSTEM IN 60 SECONDS | 126
AN ANYTIME BREATH TOOL FOR OVERWHELM
By Trish Brewer, Certified Breathwork Coach

Chapter 14
A NOURISHING BALANCE | 138
FEEL GOOD FEEDING BABY AND FUELING YOUR BODY
By Beth Conlon, PhD, RDN

Chapter 15
PLANNING AHEAD WITH YOUR ESTATE PLANNING | 151
CREATING A PLAN FOR YOUR FAMILY
By Valerie E. Anias, Esq., Founder of A Team Family Law, LLC

Chapter 16
SWEEPING AWAY CHAOS | 161
SIMPLE STEPS TO KEEP YOUR SPACE CLEAN AND ORGANIZED
By Kaitlyn Martin and Shelly Schoff, Co-Owners of Crabtown Cleaning

---

Chapter 17
REPLENISHING WHOLENESS | 172
RESTORING THE MIND, BODY, AND SOUL CONNECTION AFTER CHILDBIRTH
By Dr. Irum Tahir

Chapter 18
EMBRACING IMPERFECTION | 181
REDISCOVERING BODY CONFIDENCE AFTER CHILDBIRTH
By Tara De Leon, MS, RSCC, CSCS*D, Author, Speaker, Mama

CLOSING CHAPTER | 190

ACKNOWLEDGMENTS | 195

Introduction

JULY 11, 2021

It was the morning of my son's first birthday. Against my better judgment, we were having a party for him. Because of the pandemic, we didn't get to do a real baby shower, maternity pictures, or anything like that, so I wanted to make sure we didn't miss out on even more important events now that he was here. So, a first birthday party was happening. After prepping all morning, making sure everything was perfect—okay, okay, as good as it could be with a one-year-old running around—I quickly hopped in the shower, hoping to be fully clothed by the time guests started arriving.

The hot water ran down my body, but I barely noticed it.

Where am I going to put the food? Ugh, add body wash to the shopping list. Did I buy enough plates? Wait, is the caterer bringing plates?

I hope nobody gets COVID. Should I cancel it? Too late now.

I can't believe the baker misspelled his name on the cake. Sigh. *Nothing we can do about it at this point. Maybe I'll laugh about it someday.*

Looking down at my body, I realize it doesn't look like it used to. *That's okay. I grew and birthed an entire human, after all. This body has done some amazing things.*

Then I notice my legs. *Oh my gosh! Girl! When was the last time you shaved your legs? Weeks? Has it actually been months? Holy smokes, sis, you have got to get your shizz together. Your son is a year old. How did that time go by so fast? And you're still over here acting like you just had him!*

It was then that I knew. I was a hot mess.

I still wore nursing clothes, even though that journey ended months before. *But they're so comfy.* I still felt like I didn't have anything figured out. *Everyone else seems to have it all together.* I didn't know where to start to get things figured out. My childcare situation was less than ideal. The guilt of even having an outside caregiver for my son during a global pandemic was gnawing at me.

Should I stay home with him? I like my lifestyle now. And I love my job. I don't want to give that up. Does that make me selfish? Or worse, a bad mom?

And don't even get me started on my exercise routine. As a personal trainer, I've always enjoyed moving my body and loved working out during pregnancy. But since I had my son, I just couldn't figure out where to fit it in, not to mention cooking healthy foods. Or like any food that wasn't carryout.

Yikes.

My relationships all changed. Not necessarily for better or worse, just different. My husband and I had less time for date nights (not that many restaurants were open anyway). We were still trying to socially distance so hanging with friends and family wasn't as frequent. As introverted as I am, my cup wasn't being filled. And my husband, the extrovert? His cup was empty.

Hope I can fill those up again someday.

My libido? Gone. My anxiety? Way up. My doctor? Completely indifferent. "Welcome to motherhood," she said. "Anxiety comes with the territory, and your libido might come back once he goes to college." She paused, "Wait, how old are you?" *Checks notes* "No, you'll be in menopause by then, so it's probably gone."

Great.

As I chatted with friends (and by "chatted with friends," I mean we sent memes and videos to each other on Instagram), I realized this story was too common. Many of us, me included, went through years of trying to get pregnant, followed by fertility treatments, and then eventually having our babies. We had all the feelings: Sadness. Confusion. Fear. Hope. Optimism. Joy. Happiness. Jealousy. Anticipation. Excitement. Pregnant or not? Healthy or not? Boy or Girl? There was a lot going on there, and before we knew it, we were mamas. Well, for me, it took five years, but somehow, it still feels like "before I knew it."

I focused on getting pregnant and then actually being pregnant, for so long that I almost forgot who I was. Did you know that elephants are pregnant for 22 months? They say an elephant never forgets, but I'm guessing that after being pregnant for 22 freaking months, she can't even remember a time before she was pregnant, let alone who she was back then. Throw in the stressor of a global pandemic, and who even was I?

As I stood there in the shower, listening to the toddler banging on the door, making another mental note about needing to repaint the ceiling again, and trying to be grateful for the little things like a hot shower, I thought about the mother I wanted to be and what kind of mother my son deserved. I concluded that I wanted to be HOT: Healthy, on it, and thriving.

Health has always been important to me. I want to feel good in my body and to have my body perform the way I want it to. I'm not asking for miracles here. I wanted to be healthy enough to be able to watch my son grow up, get up and down off the floor easily, and have enough stamina to keep up with him. I'm not competing in sports or bodybuilding, etc. I just want to be healthy, regardless of how my body looks.

Being "on it" is important to me, too. I like working and staying organized, and I feel better about my entire life when I have my life together-ish. Do I have some of those little things done that you need to do when you have a baby, like estate planning and saving for the future? *At least I set up that college savings plan, but I really gotta get on the rest of it.* Am I keeping up with life's little tasks? *On a good day, kind of.* Except for laundry, because honestly, who can keep up with that? It's like the never-ending story of motherhood.

And thriving speaks to my happiness. I ask myself questions like: Am I happy? Is my son thriving? Are my relationships fulfilling? Do I have a social life? Am I excelling at work? Do I have any hobbies? Do I get to travel or do things that I want, just for me?

From that moment, the seed of this book was planted. I was a hot mess, but I wanted to become a H.O.T. mom. If I wanted to be like this, surely other moms would want this too, right? And how easy would it be if I had a checklist of tools I could use to help me get there?

So, thank you for trusting me with part of your postpartum journey. I know it's so stressful figuring out how to get out of the hot mess stage. I know you don't feel like yourself. And I know you are *thrilled* to be a mama. And that you can't imagine ever loving anyone or anything as much as you love that little angel over there. But somehow, you don't feel exactly like yourself. In so many ways, it is *so much better*. But also, you might also feel like you lost a little of yourself.

Girl, you deserve to feel like you again. You deserve to thrive at this mama thing. I have curated a panel of incredible experts, many of whom helped me personally in my journey through early motherhood. From getting my sexy back, healing my pelvic floor to stop the dreaded "pee-sneeze," feeding my baby, nourishing myself, creating a safe sleep environment for my son, making sure I was sleeping too, learning to manage my time differently, monitoring my mental health, and making my home a more zen space - even with all the extra baby items around, these women are incredible and have so much to offer. Much of their guidance changed the way I live my life. I hope that it will enhance your life too. So read this book, apply what suits you, and go thrive as a hot mom!

Xoxo,

Tara

CHAPTER 1

Rebuilding Strength

GENTLE EXERCISES FOR POSTPARTUM RECOVERY

Tara De Leon, MS, RSCC, CSCS*D, Speaker, Mama

MY STORY

My love story begins with hate. I hated my body. I got a terrible haircut for my super thick hair. My teeth were crooked. I was uncoordinated. And, worst of all, I was fat. When I was a kid, I was taller than everyone in my class, bigger than everyone my age, and all I wanted to do was blend in. A smaller body would've helped with that.

I was so obsessed with what my body looked like that I didn't even care what it could do. *What size am I? Does my belly poke out over the top of my jeans? Can I see my ribs? Am I skinnier than my friends? Do I deserve that food? Did I earn it today? Can I stand to go without it?*

I hopped on the scale every day after school, and the number shown there either made or broke my day. It was one of those old-timey scales, black metal with the weights you had to slide at the top. I left the weights exactly where they were from the day before, praying I'd be able to tap it just a hair to the left. I even began stripping off all my clothes before stepping on the scale, even though it was in the kitchen near a big bay window and a glass French door. Moving that little weight over was of utmost importance. Being skinny was an all-consuming thought.

This probably seems crazy or maybe even sad to you, but honestly, this was how it was in the 90s. Thin was in. Kate Moss hit the fashion scene, and we all wanted her look. "Nothing tastes as good as skinny feels," she proclaimed. Obviously, she has never eaten a piece of Junior's Cheesecake, or she would never say something so ridiculous. Of course, this was unfortunate for me since I've always had a sizable backside. Sir-Mix-A-Lot did his part to end America's obsession with thinness by releasing "Baby Got Back," and later, Jennifer Lopez and her booty made their debut. JLo was (and still is) gorgeous and sassy, although, according to Chris Rock, she had "a butt so big, it needs its own limousine." I started re-evaluating my body. *Maybe I'll never look like Kate, but is Jennifer a possibility?*

It was right around this time that my life-long love affair began. Who finds their true love while in high school? Me. In more than one way, me. I actually did meet my husband in high school, but that's not what we're talking about here. Yes, this torrid love affair started for all the wrong reasons but ultimately led me down a life-changing path. It was like sneaking around with that bad boy, the good-looking one, the one you knew was such a bad influence but was oh-so-fun and exciting. The one your parents hated, but you were drawn to, like a moth to the flame, and you couldn't stay away.

I'd skip school to go see him. I'd stay out late, working up a sweat. Nights, weekends, and sometimes even an early morning sweat sesh before school. Things were getting pretty serious. I wanted to bring my friends around to meet him, but nobody ever wanted to go. They didn't understand what I saw in him. "You're always spending time with him," they complained. "I can't believe you're skipping fun stuff to hang out with him."

His name? Gym. Gold's Gym.

Gold's Gym was the grungiest gym Annapolis, Maryland had to offer. It was full of meathead dude-bros who had all the fitness secrets I craved; it was love at first sight. I finally found the place that would help me sculpt, tone, and beat my body into submission, achieving the figure I always wanted. When I joined the gym, they told me I'd get two free sessions with a personal trainer. *Yes! I'll get to pick a knowledgeable trainer's brain about what I need to be doing to finally lose the weight and probably become a Victoria's Secret model.* Never mind that I was only 5'3".

At my first session with my assigned trainer—this thin, toned, tan fitness goddess—I showed up wearing stiletto heels, leather pants, and a sequined shirt. I looked like I would've been more at home in a club than in a gym. Also, leather pants? Why were those ever even a thing? They're unforgiving and uncomfortable, and God forbid if you ever sweat in them. Much like Ross from Friends, you'll never get them back on if you do. I have no idea why I wore that outfit, but somehow, that seemed like appropriate gym attire to the 17-year-old me, so that's what I wore.

This trainer took one look at me and thought for sure that she was wasting her time. Little did she know, I hated my body enough that I'd have spent my entire meager hostessing paycheck on her services without hesitation. She walked me around the gym, pointing out various machines that all promised to firm, tighten, and enhance my body. "This one is for your butt," she explained. "That one does your inner thighs, that one the back of your arms."

I was bursting with excitement and hope. This is where the magic happens! Of course, I was right, but for all the wrong reasons. I threw myself into exercising with an excitement usually reserved for 'NSYNC concerts. I spent all my free time there. I took classes: kickboxing, spinning, boot camp, anything to burn calories, oftentimes two in a row.

I worked hard in that quest to shrink myself, and honestly, I didn't notice much shrinking happening. It was disappointing, but I kept at it, hoping that eventually, it would pay off and I'd have the body of my dreams. At Sam's Club with my mom one day, she asked me to throw a case of water into the cart. I walked over and picked it up with no problem at all. *Huh. That's kind of awesome. Not skinny but strong. I'll take it—for now.*

Later in college, I enrolled in a class called "Sports Fitness Techniques." I thought it was a workout class that would help me stave off the dreaded Freshman 15. Turns out, it was a class for coaching majors, which I was not, but my professor was so passionate that I was hooked. He taught us squats, deadlifts, power cleans, snatches, and more. The thing that really caught my attention was the Karvonen formula for the target training zone. Basically, this was like the cheat code for burning fat at all times, or so I thought. I spent hours on the elliptical, diligently staying in my target training zone, hoping to burn those calories.

I started to realize that being strong was awesome and empowering. *Who cares if I'm not super thin if I can be badass? Why be a model when I can be a superhero?* As I let this idea start to marinate, someone told me I should be a personal trainer. *Oh. Hell. Yeah. I will learn how to finally get what I want! This will be the perfect way to get paid to exercise, and all personal trainers are fit, so yay! This is it! And wearing Nikes and workout clothes every day? I am so down.*

Turns out that you don't actually get paid to exercise as a trainer. You're so busy critiquing your client's form that you don't have time to worry about yourself. But by the time I realized that I was in and loving it! I worked with all types of clients, from athletes to old ladies, businessmen to stay-at-home moms, pregnant women to women in menopause, kids to teens, and everything in between. One-on-one or in small groups, in large groups or huge groups. Fitness was my jam, and I owned it. It became a part of my identity. To this day, my friends and family ask why I'm "so fancy" if I'm in regular shoes and jeans. Seeing me in tennis shoes and leggings is how you'll usually find me.

I switched my major to exercise and sports science, got my Master's Degree in kinesiology, and studied for and achieved a ton of certifications on the way. After graduate school, I started to notice that I didn't really have that drive to be skinny anymore. The hate was gone. I threw out my scale and started to train to be strong, confident, and badass instead. Worrying about the number of pounds on the scale was way less interesting than worrying about the number of pounds on the bar.

I leaned into this. It felt so much better than being insecure all the time. I shifted my focus at work from clients who wanted to be thin to clients who wanted to feel good about themselves and their bodies to feel good. My client book exploded. It seemed like everyone just needed permission to say, "Hey, I'm good the way I am. I don't need to shrink. I have value no matter what size my jeans are. My weight is the least interesting thing about me."

Breaking up with exercising for the wrong reasons was one of the nicest things I've ever done for myself and my clients. Like that toxic love affair, every now and then, that bad boy tries to weasel his way back into my life, but now I have the skills to recognize that diet culture for what it is and the tools to tell him that it's over. We're through, and I never want to see his face ever again.

For years, I practiced exercising for the right reasons. I found my true calling. Then, as life tends to do, a wrench was thrown in that changed my body and my expectations around exercise. After years of trying, lots of fertility treatments, surgery, and a miscarriage, I eventually got pregnant. I kept exercising throughout my pregnancy and felt so healthy and happy. Once I had my son, I was sure I'd be able to jump right back into lifting and working out.

Not so fast. Even with an easy pregnancy, aside from trouble conceiving, being geriatric and obese (those were the doctor's words, not mine. Mine would have been more like healthy, happy, and strong), not the greatest time in labor, and an unplanned NICU stay (if you want to hear that crazy story, I did a podcast episode on it. Listen here: https://podcasts.apple.com/us/podcast/wellness-rebranded-intuitive-eating-diet-culture-food/id1651744916) I just knew I'd be okay exercising right away.

I was not. Nothing felt quite right. Nothing hurt, but it wasn't normal. Walking was okay, so I did that for short distances, but any sort of lifting, my love language, my identity, didn't feel good.

Well, this is unexpected. How could I have been lifting and crushing it like a month ago and now feel like my entire core is gone? Is my entire pelvic floor falling out?

Well, hello! You just grew an entire human, birthed him, and are now recovering from that! Things moved around in there; it'll get better; give it time.

After six months, I saw my doctor. "I keep peeing my pants every time I sneeze," I complained. "Should I see a pelvic floor physical therapist?" I asked. "If you want to, but it might not help," she replied. I decided to try physical therapy and find a new doctor.

Pelvic floor physical therapy was life-changing for me. After just a few sessions, I felt stronger and more like myself than I'd felt in a long time. I was able to get back to training but recognized that the demands on my time had changed. I only had 20-30 minutes, usually. Sometimes, I didn't even have time to get to the gym, so home workouts became more common. Moving my body in a way that made me feel good was the priority. I didn't want to come home exhausted. I wanted to move well and feel rejuvenated so I could take on all the tasks of new mamahood and still feel like myself.

That's exactly what I did. I studied for specialty certifications dealing with pregnancy and postpartum, and I created an awesome workout for myself to help me feel good in my body and improve my mental and physical wellness. In the coming pages, I provide a tool for you to add to your tool kit as you begin your own postpartum journey. Returning to exercise, or even starting exercise for the first time, can be intimidating, but I'm here to help. I know you want to be the healthiest version of yourself to care for that baby and then watch that baby grow up. This tool will get you started the right way on that journey. We got this!

THE TOOL

I didn't start truly weightlifting again until about 24 weeks postpartum. Talk to your doctor about starting a gentle exercise program, but don't push it yet. There will be time for that later, but for right now, we just need to heal and move a little bit. Listen to your body! If things aren't feeling great for you at eight weeks postpartum, please wait until you're feeling better or talk to a professional (*Hi! It's me! Or a physical therapist, or your doc*) about getting started. We want this to enhance your life, not hinder it.

Return to Exercise Training Program

Timeframe: 8-18 weeks postpartum

Goals: Rest, recovery, maintaining good breathing patterns and good core and pelvic floor coordination while incorporating some strength training exercises.

Equipment: If you're doing this at a gym, great. You'll have everything you need. If you are doing this at home, buy a set of bands with handles and some 5, 10, and 15-pound dumbbells. If you can get a pair of adjustable dumbbells, that would be ideal because then you won't outgrow the plan for a long time.

Note: For these workouts, you'll pick two days a week to do the strength training, at least two days apart, and then cycle through them. For example, if you're lifting on Tuesdays and Thursdays, you'll do Workout A on Tuesday, Workout B on Thursday, and Workout C the following Tuesday. If your body is feeling good, feel free to do them three days a week, but no more than that. Rest and recovery are key during this postpartum period.

HOT MESS TO HOT MOM POSTPARTUM WORKOUT

8–12 WEEKS POSTPARTUM

WARM UP	Connection Breath	1 x 10 Breaths
	Cardio Warm-Up	5 minutes
STRENGTH TRAINING	Full-body strength training sessions	Two or three days per week
CARDIO	Walk	No more than 45 minutes per day at an easy pace as often as you are comfortable
REST AND RECOVERY	Rest as much as possible throughout the day.	

STRENGTH TRAINING WORKOUT A

EXERCISE	WEEKS 8-9	WEEKS 10-12	REST
1A. BODYWEIGHT SQUAT	3 x 10-12	3-4 x 8-10	30 seconds
1B. LAT PULLDOWN	3 x 10-12	3-4 x 8-10	60 seconds
2A. SINGLE LEG ROMANIAN DEADLIFT	3 x 8	3-4 x 8	30 seconds
2B. HIGH INCLINE PUSHUP	3 x 10-12	3-4 x 8-10	30 seconds
2C. PALLOFF PRESS	3 x 10-12	3-4 x 8-10	60 seconds

STRENGTH TRAINING WORKOUT B

EXERCISE	WEEKS 8-9	WEEKS 10-12	REST
1A. ROMANIAN DEADLIFT	3 x 10-12	3-4 x 8-10	30 seconds
1B. BANDED ROW	3 x 10-12	3-4 x 8-10	30 seconds
2A. REVERSE LUNGE	3 x 10-12	3-4 x 8-10	30 seconds
2B. SHOULDER PRESS	3 x 10-12	3-4 x 8-10	30 seconds
2C. SIDE PLANK	3 x 15 seconds	3-4 x 15-20 seconds	30 seconds

STRENGTH TRAINING WORKOUT C

EXERCISE	WEEKS 8-9	WEEKS 10-12	REST
1A. GLUTE BRIDGE	3 x 10-12	3-4 x 8-10	30 seconds
1B. SINGLE ARM DUMBBELL ROW	3 x 10-12	3-4 x 8-10	30 seconds
2A. DUMBBELL BENCH PRESS	3 x 10-12	3-4 x 8-10	30 seconds
2B. BIRD DOG	3 x 15 seconds	3-4 x 15-20 seconds	30 seconds
2C. LATERAL LUNGE	3 x 10-12	3-4 x 8-10	30 seconds

13-18 WEEKS POSTPARTUM

If you don't start exercising again at eight weeks, go back and do the first part of this workout no matter how far postpartum you are. Don't worry that the weeks won't match up for you; it's what your body needs. Then, once you've done that for four weeks, come back to this point.

WARM UP	Connection Breath	1 x 10 Breaths
	Cardio Warm-Up	5 minutes
STRENGTH TRAINING	Full-body strength training sessions	Two to three days per week
CARDIO	Walk	Up to 60 minutes a day at an easy pace as often as you are comfortable.
	Moderate Intensity Cardio	If you feel up for it, you can ease back into one moderate-intensity cardio session per week for 15-30 minutes. If you feel up for it, you can ease back into one high-intensity cardio session per week for 8-10 minutes.
	High-Intensity Cardio	
REST AND RECOVERY	You should rest as much as possible throughout the day.	

STRENGTH TRAINING WORKOUT A

EXERCISE	WEEKS 13-15	WEEKS 16-18	REST
1A. GOBLET SQUAT	3 x 8-10	3-4 x 10-12	30 seconds
1B. FACE PULL	3 x 8-10	3-4 x 10-12	30 seconds
2A. STEP UPS	3 x 8-10	3-4 x 10-12	30 seconds
2B. INCLINE PUSHUPS	3 x 8-10	3-4 x 10-12	30 seconds
3A. SPLIT SQUAT	3 x 8-10	3-4 x 10-12	30 seconds
3B. PALLOFF PRESSES	3 x 8-10	3-4 x 10-12	30 seconds

STRENGTH TRAINING WORKOUT B

EXERCISE	WEEKS 13-15	WEEKS 16-18	REST
1A. HIP THRUST	3 x 8-10	3-4 x 10-12	30 seconds
1B. HALF KNEELING BAND ROW	3 x 8-10	3-4 x 10-12	60 seconds
2A. CURTSY LUNGE	3 x 8-10	3-4 x 10-12	30 seconds
2B. LATERAL RAISE	3 x 8-10	3-4 x 10-12	60 seconds
3A. BICEPS CURLS	3 x 8-10	3-4 x 10-12	30 seconds
3B. TRICEPS PUSHDOWNS	3 x 8-10	3-4 x 10-12	60 seconds

STRENGTH TRAINING WORKOUT C

EXERCISE	WEEKS 13-15	WEEKS 16-18	REST
1A. ROMANIAN DEADLIFT	3 x 8-10	3-4 x 10-12	30 seconds
1B. SINGLE ARM DUMBBELL ROW	3 x 8-10	3-4 x 10-12	60 seconds
2A. SINGLE LEG GLUTE BRIDGE	3 x 8-10	3-4 x 10-12	30 seconds
2B. BODYWEIGHT WALKING LUNGES	3 x 8-10	3-4 x 10-12	60 seconds
3A. HAMMER CURLS	3 x 8-10	3-4 x 10-12	30 seconds
3B. PALLOFF PRESS	3 x 8-10	3-4 x 10-12	60 seconds

*Note: The Connection Breath is arguably the most important part of this workout. Start in whatever position you like. Inhale, and relax the pelvic floor. This will feel like the muscles you would use to stop the flow of urine. On exhale, lift it upwards.

If you would like to download this workout on my custom app, which has cues and videos of each exercise, go to this link: http://bit.ly/HotMesstoHotMom.

As much as I love exercising and lifting weights, if you're having back, pelvic, or tailbone pain that lasts more than two weeks after delivery, you need to wait. Any pain, numbness, or tingling in your hips or legs, or if you have diastasis recti (a separation of your abdominal muscles) are also good reasons to wait. If you're experiencing these symptoms, I would recommend talking to a physical therapist. I'm a huge fan of pelvic floor physical therapy and think all new moms should have at least a consult postpartum, especially if you're experiencing those symptoms.

A note to all the C-section mamas out there. Be gentle with yourself. Not only did you just grow an entire human, but you also had your body cut open. You can still do these workouts, starting at eight weeks, but please be extra mindful about pain. You should not have any pain while exercising, and if you feel any tugging or pulling on your scar, skip that exercise for now.

I would LOVE to hear from you! If you start doing this workout and have any questions, please don't hesitate to reach out to me.

Healing from birth is no joke. Your body doesn't define your self-worth, and exercising can be a celebration of what it can do. Be proud of what your body just accomplished and remember that your body has just given you one of the greatest gifts of your life - your child.

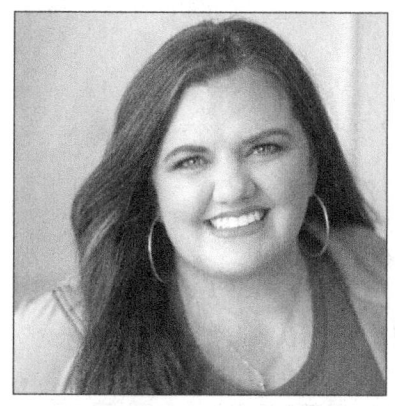

Tara De Leon is a personal trainer, professor of Health, Fitness and Exercise Studies, podcaster, speaker, and author. Tara has helped hundreds of women feel badass and confident by teaching them how to lift weights and get strong, healthy, and empowered. Tara teaches women to take up space and to stop apologizing for their bodies. Specializing in fitness for fertility, prenatal and postnatal fitness, she loves helping moms go from hot mess to hot mom. Tara is passionate about health and fitness and strives to constantly improve herself to better help her clients.

Tara has a master's degree in Human Movement from A.T. Still University of Health Sciences, a bachelor's degree in Exercise and Sports Science from Brigham Young University-Hawaii, and maintains 14 other advanced certifications pertaining to fitness, wellness, and lifestyle. She has won "Best Personal Trainer" twice, "Best Lifestyle Coach" once, and has been voted "Best Prenatal Fitness Coach" four years in a row by What's Up Annapolis Magazine. She is a nominee for Personal Trainer of the Year by the National Strength and Conditioning Association.

When Tara is not working, you can find her eating sushi or tacos, going for walks, baking, and spending time on the Chesapeake Bay with her husband, Marcus, their 3-year-old son, Maverick, and their Aussie pup, Chula.

If you are interested in working with Tara, reach out to set up a free consultation. She would love to help you thrive as the HOT mom that you are.

Tara De Leon
TaraRDeLeon@gmail.com
Instagram: @Tara_De_Leon_Fitness
Facebook: @TaraDeLeonFitness
Website: ptdistinction.com/TaraDeLeonFitness
Podcast: Wellness Rebranded

CHAPTER 2

Restless to Restful

SIMPLE STEPS FOR MOMS TO GET GREAT SLEEP

Kelly Myerson, MA, OTR

MY STORY

"Silent night, holy night. All is calm; all is bright," I sang quietly as I looked down at the sleepy-faced babe in my arms. The dim lights of the Christmas tree cast a warm glow in the living room.

My little guy stopped nursing, and I hummed the tune as I switched him to the other side to finish.

"You like the Christmas tree, don't you, little one," I sweetly whispered to him.

He paused nursing long enough to look up at me and smile a toothless smile. Then he resumed.

"Me too, buddy."

I sighed, "Silent night, holy night. Shepherds quake at the sight." As his breathing slowed, I continued humming gently, swaying from side to side.

Shifting him to my right shoulder, I adjusted my pajama top. Standing up slowly so as not to disturb him, I moved across the dining room to the stairs.

I crept up the stairs, continuing my humming as we reached the landing. His nursery door was right in front of us.

I smiled to myself, pleased I had the foresight to lower the lights in his nursery and turn on the sound machine.

One gentle transfer to the crib, and it's nighty night for me, too!

Looking down at the peaceful, snuggly boy in my arms, I couldn't help but feel I had everything I could ever want this Christmas season.

A baby sigh slipped out of his mouth as he nuzzled into my chest.

I continued humming as I stood on my tippy toes to lift him over the side of the crib and lay him down gently.

He stirred for a moment, then settled back into sleep. Humming, I took slow steps to the door and closed it as I moved into the hallway.

Twenty steps, and I was at my nightstand. I switched on the monitor and briefly stared at the sleeping baby on the darkened screen. He was still. I felt tired.

Climbing into bed, I pulled the blanket up to my chin and smiled. Rolling over, I set my alarm on my phone for 6 am and laughed. "Not that I need an alarm!"

Returning my phone to the nightstand, I glanced at the time. It was 6:30 pm. My husband crept in quietly.

"He's asleep?" He whispered.

"Yup."

"And you're really going to bed now?" He gave me a puzzled look.

"Yup." I smiled at him and snuggled down deeper.

"Okay." He went on. "And you're sure it's okay if I sleep in the guest room tonight? I could use a good night of sleep."

"We all need a good night of sleep," I replied, yawning to prove the point.

"Okay, babe. I love you. Come get me if you need me in the middle of the night."

"I will. Love you too." I said as he kissed my head before walking to the door and turning off the light.

Smiling, I rolled to my left side for one more glance at the sleeping baby boy down the hall.

"Sweet dreams, little one. See you in a few hours." I chuckled, knowing our series of early morning feedings would begin around 1 am if I was lucky.

I breathed deeply and prepared to get a few good hours of sleep before he'd need to eat. I looked at the sparse bed. I'd learned to sleep with a simple blanket.

Sweet dreams, mama.

I drifted off to sleep, hearing the noise machine come through the monitor.

Awakened at 12:30 am to the sound of my baby crying, I padded down the hallway and opened the door. He was rolled on his side, looking at the door, and cried harder as I walked towards him.

Picking him up, he nuzzled my shoulder and whimpered.

"Are you hungry? Would you like to nurse?" I snuggled him close and quietly walked to my bedroom, closing the door behind us.

I laid him in the middle of the king-sized bed and climbed in next to him. I pulled him close to me once I was settled on my right side facing him.

He briefly cried but stopped as soon as he latched on. Gently stroking his head, I closed my eyes and recalled the phone conversation I'd had with my mom a couple of weeks ago.

"Mom, I'm exhausted!" I cried. "He wakes up every couple of hours to eat, and I never get to sleep! I'm going back and forth from my bedroom to his nursery all night long!"

"Kelly, this is the best advice I can give you. You should do whatever you need to do for you and the baby to get sleep."

My mom was right. I realized my sleep was so much better when I accepted that my baby needed to be near me overnight. I needed to go to bed when he did because the best stretch of sleep available to me was 6:30 pm to 12:30 am.

It was a life-changing decision to abandon my self-imposed expectations for motherhood. My baby didn't sleep through the night or easily transition back to his crib. I couldn't continue to function as a mom, a wife, or a human being in the world.

I decided to follow my mom's advice. I decided to follow my intuition. I decided to prioritize my rest and sleep first and let it be what worked for us.

Deciding was the hardest part of my shift. Taking action to focus on a bedtime routine for both of us was a matter of a few simple steps.

After dinner, he and I began our nighttime routines. I packed up my lunch for the next day, showered, got into pajamas, and set out my work clothes. He had a bath, got into his pajamas, and had a little time with my husband.

Then, it was time for my baby and I to have our time. Our breastfeeding journey wasn't as easy, so my heart always flooded with gratitude during his bedtime feedings.

Prioritizing rest and sleep gave me back a sense of self and the ability to function. I was no longer celebrating exhaustion. I was celebrating the ability to nourish not just my beautiful baby boy but *myself*. I, too, was deserving of compassion and care.

How are you, mama? If you've picked up this book and you're reading this chapter, I can imagine the level of fatigue and frustration with which you're living. If you resonate with my story, then I'm here to make it simple for you to get great sleep too. Let's take you from restless to restful.

Sleep is foundational to our health. I'd go as far as to state without adequate sleep it doesn't matter what else you do for your well-being. Lack of sleep has a critical impact on your physical, emotional, and psychological well-being.

Case in point, as a brand new mom 76 hours into motherhood, with barely any sleep, I felt like I was being tortured.

In addition to poor sleep, I struggled with postpartum anxiety and crippling perfectionism. Ten years ago, when I had my son, they asked me questions to determine if I was depressed. I wasn't. There weren't any questions about experiencing anxiety.

It wasn't just stress. I experienced full panic that at any moment, something I'd do (or not do) would result in the death of my baby. On top of that, I applied my lifetime of perfectionism to motherhood and was devastated I didn't measure up.

As a result, I pushed myself to the brink of exhaustion.

Emotional breakdowns were a regular occurrence, and without quality sleep, I was drowning. All the while, I fought to keep up with my job, pumping, breastfeeding, and providing my child with all the love he deserved.

Meanwhile, my shell of a body felt betrayed. She longed for peace and rest. For too long, I denied her. I asked her to keep going. Caring for myself felt like one more item on the growing to-do list.

Are you feeling the same way I did?

THE TOOL

Oh, mama, ten years later, my heart is breaking for you. My heart is breaking for all the moms who believe this is how it's supposed to be. I had a supportive and involved husband. I had outside support. Yet, I still couldn't reconcile how to care for my baby, my home, and me.

Luckily, you're holding the key to making decisions to change your life for the better in your hands.

Let's get you to a more restful state in your body and your mind. As a side note, I'm going to keep this simple and easy on purpose. This is a start to getting better sleep. When you're ready, I have a wealth of resources for you here: https://www.beingwellwithkelly.com/hmhmresources.

STEP 1: CHOOSE TO PRIORITIZE YOURSELF

Decide to focus on your physical needs. You deserve the same level of care and consideration you give your child at bedtime. I recommend including tasks in the evening to prepare for sleep *and* prepare for the next day. It doesn't matter if you're a stay-at-home mom or a working mom. Prepping for the next day has become the best way to care for myself. Being prepared makes me feel more restful.

STEP 2: PREPARE FOR THE NEXT DAY

Consider what kind of morning you need. Does your baby need a lot of your time? Are you not a morning person? Set out everyone's clothes for the next day and have breakfast and lunch already prepared. If, like me, you need coffee before facing the world, set it to turn on automatically when you wake up.

Take your bath or shower at night. I suggest getting yourself ready for bed before putting your baby to bed. That way when bedtime doesn't go as smoothly as you'd like, you only have to put yourself to bed after.

STEP 3: DO LESS AND SIMPLIFY EVERYTHING

If it feels overwhelming to complete all those tasks, then it's time to simplify. I aspired to be a perfect mom. That was my first mistake. The perfect mom doesn't exist, despite what we may see on social media. Most moms are just doing their best. That's good enough.

Release your ideal vision of motherhood. I envisioned a perfect pain-free, natural birth, easy breastfeeding, and a baby who slept like a dream. I envisioned making my own baby food and effortlessly keeping a clean and organized home. Oh, and I was going to look beautifully put together every day.

I learned, over time, to accept what hadn't happened the way I planned. I also accepted what was not possible for me without burning out. I focused on my baby and what he needed to function. Mostly, he needed me. He needed my presence and warmth to calm his nervous system.

Let go of the image of motherhood you're beating yourself up about. She doesn't exist. Instead, choose what to prioritize.

I chose to prioritize a daily shower and coffee every morning. I chose to prioritize getting sleep over productivity or free time in the evening. I went to bed early so I could be available to him when he needed me most. I cut out every unnecessary task.

Be ruthless with your time. This is one season. When you're in it, it feels like it'll never end. It does.

What does your baby need most from you? When do they need you most? Cultivate your routines based on their needs. Simplify them so you have time to get extra rest and sleep.

Here are some quick and easy ways to simplify. This isn't an exhaustive list. Before reading it, I'd like you to release judgment of yourself or other moms who choose shortcuts.

We're in survival mode. We need to prioritize our well-being. This isn't the time to worry about saving the environment or eating 100% organic whole foods made from scratch. In the future, when everyone sleeps regularly, and you feel like a million bucks, you can consider other values and priorities. For now, focus on your health and well-being and caring for your baby.

- Use paper plates, bowls, and plastic utensils.
- Buy premade meals and/or prepackaged foods to put in lunches.
- Batch cook when you have time and freeze meals.
- Order food. Order extra food, if you can afford it, to have for the next day or freeze for the future.
- Simplify your wardrobe. Wear clothes you can wash, dry, and wear.
- Minimize your bathing routine. Fewer products mean fewer steps.
- Delegate. Delegate to anyone you can think of in your life. Delegate household tasks to your partner, if you have one, or your other children. Delegate to your friend who's been asking what she can do for you.
- Order groceries to be delivered. Order diapers to be delivered. Delivery is your friend when it's hard to get out of your home with a baby.
- Say "no" to all invitations, opportunities, and tasks for which you don't have the time, energy, or interest.
- Say "yes" to all invitations for someone to help you.
- Let go of control. When you delegate or ask for help, let go of how someone else completes the task. Be grateful for the help and ask for it again.

- Keep play and living spaces simplified. Get baskets or containers to easily put items away by tossing them in. Put away all the extras and just have a few items out at a time so the space doesn't become overwhelmed.

STEP 4: DO WHAT WORKS FOR YOU

People will judge and comment on your choices as a mom. Let them. You do you, mama. Fearlessly choose to prioritize the well-being of you and your baby. Purposefully put you first.

My biggest lesson as a mom has been to put me first. It's revolutionary. Imagine how much we can do for our kiddos when we feel great. Start with prioritizing your rest and sleep. If you've followed these steps and sleep is still elusive, I'm here for you. Reach out to me through my resource page https://www.beingwellwithkelly.com/hmhmresources.

Weariness was a piece of motherhood I believed I couldn't escape. It's no longer my badge of honor. I no longer celebrate exhaustion. I choose me. I care for myself. I take time to rest. And, mama, I get great sleep!

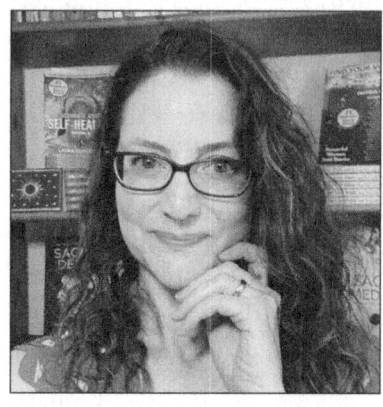

Kelly is an author, podcaster, and sleep specialist who will cultivate space for you to emerge from stress and overwhelm to lead and savor the life of your dreams. As an occupational therapist, Kelly has over 23 years of experience specializing in sensory integration techniques. Her background in occupational therapy provides a unique perspective on development and the human condition. She values personal power and inspires all of us to build our capacity to surpass our potential by living in alignment with our true selves.

With a Master's degree in Strategic Communication and Leadership, she brings data-driven techniques leading to lasting change. Over the past 17 years, she has experience teaching topics including self-care, leadership development, outcome measurement, sensory processing related to anxiety, and sleep. Kelly is a holistic entrepreneur bringing a wealth of experience and fun science to the table, whether speaking to engaging guests on The Mystic Nerd Squad Podcast or supporting women in revitalizing their lives.

You can check out her other six chapters in the Amazon Best-selling books, *Sacred Sleep: Cultivating the Best Sleep of Your Life*, in *The Ultimate Guide to Self-Healing, Volume 4*, *Courageous Self-care: Putting Myself First to Serve Others* in *Find Your Voice Save Your Life Volume 2*, *Radical Self-care for Caregivers: Nourishing Yourself Through Grief and Loss* in *Sacred Death, Sacred Rest: Be at Your Best by Doing Less* in *Sacred Medicine, Harmonize Your Divine Masculine and Feminine Energy: Get Shit Done and Feel Good Doing It* in *Wealth Codes: Sacred Strategies for Abundance,* and *Get Better in Bed: L.O.V.E. Yourself to Sleep with Foundational Habits* in Holistic Mental Health. All available at https://beingwellwithkelly.com/books/.

For additional resources related to Kelly's healing journey and to connect with her, please visit https://www.beingwellwithkelly.com.

CHAPTER 3

Running Strong: Navigating your Mother Runner Pace

AN EMPOWERED APPROACH TO SAFELY RUN POSTPARTUM

Melissa Szurovy, RRCA Certified Run Coach

MY STORY

When I inquired about joining the Naval Reserve Officers Training Corps (NROTC) the summer before my freshman year at Penn State University, I was told I needed to run a mile and a half in 15 minutes.

I thought, *I can do that*, so I figured, *why not give it a try?*

I had not participated in organized athletics since I was 13 years old, but I first started running as a teenager to lose weight. I wasn't fast. But it was the thing to do in the late 1990s.

That first physical training (PT) session at 0530 on a Tuesday in September 1999 was an eye-opener. We did a formation run where you are to stay in ranks. I fell out of ranks within the first half mile and found out it was possible to vomit from physical activity.

Whoa, these people are all very fast. I will never keep up! That was a recurring thought I had often during that first year in the NROTC program. After falling out of that first battalion run, you would've never guessed I'd end up being a running coach.

And that's just the beginning of my running journey.

I have already mentioned I wasn't fast compared to all of those other college students. To not be assigned remedial PT, I had to run the mile and a half in 13:30 minutes, not 15 minutes!

Remedial PT it was! However, since I was 18 and a novice runner, I saw progress rather quickly. And *that* is where it started.

I ran throughout college mostly to stay off of remedial PT and sometimes with other midshipmen on weekend adventures. We only got lost once! I recall knowing one fellow midshipman who ran marathons. For real, and for fun! What? I had no idea running could be fun.

After graduating from college, commissioning in the Navy, and heading to graduate school in Monterey, California, I made a new running friend. And she introduced me to my very first race—the inaugural Big Sur Half Marathon.

I was bitten by the race bug! That race made me realize I could go the distance!

Half marathons became my jam. I ran one or two a year for the next several years, and after another cross-country move and three deployments, I finally got to shore duty, where I trained and completed my first full—the Marine Corps Marathon.

One common theme my athletes come to me with is, "I didn't perform as well as I would have liked on my last race." I, too, was plagued with this thought and wondered, *what can I do next?* And *how can I do better?* after the marathon.

That aggressive downloaded plan, which was not followed religiously, left me with a nagging knee injury afterward. After rehabbing my knee, I was set to move again, returning to sea duty, with a year of various schools in three different states, including another cross-country move to San Diego.

I researched running by this point for personal knowledge. I knew I only had time to safely train up to the half marathon distance with the demanding work schedule of being on sea duty and with a deployment shortly after reporting onboard.

Upon return, I ran three half marathons in seven months. I expected this to have had me at my thinnest, but the opposite was true. All that running, with little strength training made my body good at running long distances, aka storing body fat. After consulting with a fitness expert at my command, he suggested heavy lifting. Not the 10-pound and 20-pound kettlebells I was using.

I searched Amazon and found a book. I knew if I was going to lift heavier, I needed to do it with proper form. The author of the book taught in San Deigo County! I set up a session and started attending her classes when the ship's schedule permitted.

That next Physical Readiness Test (PRT) after finding kettlebells was a personal best!

My love of kettlebells was ignited.

Now, I have two loves: Running and strength.

Duty called again, deployment and another cross-country move. This time for good. We settled in Annapolis, Maryland, and chose to start our family.

Doing some simple math and reading regulations, I'd have approximately 11 months from birth until I had to complete a PRT again. I came across an online trainer who focused on pregnant and postpartum women, including running.

I implemented her program and worked on my pelvic floor and core during pregnancy and afterward.

Unfortunately, there was external pressure to return my body to PRT standards after pregnancy. While this is not a practice I condone for the general public, I was not the general public, but I wanted to do it as safely as possible.

For the record, I smoked my 18-year-old time requirement by about 90 seconds, 15-plus years later—thank you, kettlebells!

This is where I think you'll resonate with me—during my second pregnancy. I was pregnant with my son one year after giving birth to my daughter.

I didn't have any obvious issues with my pelvic floor, but I was well aware that this second pregnancy would be different.

I was working full time, carrying a one-year-old around while growing a baby, and my pelvic floor took the brunt of the load. By the time I was in my second trimester, I couldn't sneeze without peeing my pants, and the pubic symphysis pain significantly slowed me down.

Running was the last thing on my mind at this point. Between having a toddler who thought sleep was an option, being pregnant, and the pain of just walking, I prioritized my pelvic floor work during this pregnancy.

Besides the eviction notice my son received and still taking more than 12 hours to arrive, his birth was rather uneventful. But when I went to my six-week postpartum check-up, I knew my pelvic floor didn't feel right. Heaviness, pressure, and urinary leakage were my main symptoms.

I requested a pelvic floor physical therapist (PFPT) referral. That PRT would come again, and this time, I had symptoms to manage. Thankfully, I had 14 months to prepare.

Oh, the gift of time!

After being cleared from the PFPT, I started gently running again. I was 12 weeks postpartum with my second child, the weather was beautiful, and I could just go out there and enjoy springtime running in Annapolis.

With this gift of time, I had a new approach. I wanted to enjoy every one of my runs. What did I do differently? The *instant* I felt leakage or had *any* pressure in my pelvic floor, my run was done.

This was what I refer to as the SHIFT in my relationship with running.

Having the time to slowly return to running, two to three times per week, but only if my body agreed, allowed me the freedom to run without the pressure of external goals. No pun intended! During this season, I jauntily referred to myself as a "fair-weather runner."

I had the freedom to run when I wanted to, for however long I wanted to, without being hamstrung by a specific plan or race schedule.

And most importantly, I had the knowledge and freedom to know I could stop any time my body told me it had enough and it would be just fine. And it was.

Running for fun was back!

I didn't set out to be a running coach. I set out to help other women get strong.

Little did I know how that would turn out!

I did want to help women get strong, and in the process, I found my passion for helping *mother runners get stronger*.

In the early days of the pandemic, I *needed* to get out and run. Fresh air and away from the quarantine mentality for just 20-30 minutes, with a three-year-old and five-year-old at home, all day, every day.

It dawned on me others may need this too. I polled my online strength community. They did need it! The StrongMom RunClub was born! It was a virtual community of mother runners who came together when the world was keeping everyone apart. We had weekly goal-setting, virtual meet-ups, and monthly challenges.

Throughout that summer, I ran in the blistering heat.

The following winter, I ran in the cold.

I was no longer a fair-weather runner.

I was a runner.

I *mom* better when I run.

I *wife* better when I run.

I *me* better when I run.

I am a runner.

So many moms out there run but still don't feel confident calling themself a runner. It's time to change!

As the StrongMom RunClub community grew, I realized I could combine my passion for helping women get stronger with my knowledge, coaching ability, and teaching skills.

I took that seriously.

I earned my certification as a running coach and certified personal trainer. I continue to educate myself through courses and reviewing research. I have recently discovered the lack of research on women and young athletes. I'm specifically interested in the development of our youth, not solely for their current performance, but for them to continue to love being active throughout their entire lifetime. Parents' participation in physical activity has been associated with their children's physical activity.[1]

I was texting with one of my athletes the other day. I hadn't heard from her for about a month. During our conversation, she sent this:

"I need to resign from run club. I suck."

I felt like I failed. I never want any of my athletes to feel like they suck!

I wasn't sure how to respond. I took a minute or two. This athlete has become a friend. And I know she has a goal to run a full marathon.

She is a mom of three young kiddos, has a full-time job, and I know how hard it is to do all.the.things!

I finally responded, "Do you *want* to run?"

The last thing I want is for my athletes to feel pressure to run. *There's that "p" word again.* Ultimately, the conversation is still ongoing at the time of this writing, she acknowledges she still has a marathon goal but hasn't been in a place to prioritize it. She has to want it. And want it now to effectively make it a priority. And if it isn't a right-now thing?

That is 100% completely okay.

That brings me back to you, mama.

You're itching to get back out there. You're feeling the pressure.

Only you know what your "pressure" is. I can hypothesize that it's either the fastest way to get your pre-baby body back, you want to reach a personal best race time you were chasing just before you found out you were expecting, you're overwhelmed with the laundry and dishes and diapers and *need* a break, or, oh gosh, it could be so many more things.

---

[1] Kristine A. Madsen, M.D., M.P.H., Charles McCulloch, PhD, and Patricia B. Crawford, DrPH, Parent Modeling: Perceptions of Parents' Physical Activity Predict Girls' Activity throughout Adolescence, https://www.ncbi.nlm.nih.gov/pmc/articles/PMC2654401/.

What I want you to take from this is you deserve the gift of time. Remove whatever pressure, *that p-word again*, you're under that makes you think you need to get back out there for a daily 5k or a marathon at six months postpartum.

Your body has been through a lot with pregnancy and birth and now motherhood.

Give it the time it needs to heal.

Build your running strength back up, take it easy, and please promise me that if you pee your pants when running, even if just a little, you'll stop and call your Pelvic Floor Physical Therapist.

The final statement I'd like to leave you with is this:

When I took away the pressure to meet goals that didn't have a driving purpose in my overall life, such as paces, race personal records, or PRT scores, I was able to realize how much I love running.

I want you to love running, too.

THE TOOL

AN EMPOWERED APPROACH TO SAFELY RUN POSTPARTUM

If you're reading this chapter in this book, I'm assuming you are eager to get back out in your running shoes after having a baby.

I get it; I was too! But I can tell you that too many moms go back out too soon, too often, and too fast.

That's where injuries, overtraining, and under-recovering can come back to derail you once again.

Don't be that mom. Below is an empowering guide with seven steps to get you back to running postpartum safely. And remember, I give you the gift of time.

For a printable flowchart, go to www.chesapeakerunningacademy.com/return2run

Whether you ran before the baby or you want to start now, I want you to go through this checklist first. And be honest. Judgment-free zone here.

1. DOES RUNNING BRING YOU JOY RIGHT NOW?

YES! - Go to Step 2.

Not a "Yes!"? Stop, earmark this page, and come back to this when it is. Remember, running should be fun.

2. HAVE YOU BEEN MEDICALLY CLEARED FOR HIGH-IMPACT TRAINING, INCLUDING RUNNING?

YES - This return to running will be a gradual process. Just because you ran a 5k a week before your baby's birth, or you ran a marathon six weeks pregnant, does NOT mean you can jump right back in. Go to Step 3.

NO - It's okay, mama. It takes time. Every body is different and heals differently. Remember, you're giving yourself time to navigate this postpartum era. Come back when you're ready; the roads aren't going anywhere.

Warning: This is not solely that six-week postpartum checkup. I highly recommend seeking out a pelvic floor physical therapist before starting *any* high-impact activity, especially when resuming after pregnancy.

3. ARE YOU GETTING "GOOD" SLEEP?

YES - 7-9 hours, 6-7 nights a week. Go to Step 4.

NO - You're not getting a good night's sleep? *Proceed with caution.*

Sleep is one of your best recovery tools[2] and if your baby, three-year-old, or eight-year-old is getting up most nights and/or your sleep is disrupted, you will not have optimal recovery, and it can lead to injuries. You may have just read about this in Chapter 2 by Kelly Myerson.

For the record, I want to tell you to stop. Do some walking/gentle yoga/low-impact movement until your sleep routine is better. But I know you may not heed that advice. It was hard for me to follow too.

4. ACTION TIME.

Let's try a run, run/walk. Start with ten minutes total. A 1:1 ratio of run/walking, such as 60-second run and 60-second walk intervals, is a good start. Adjust the ratio as your body tells you. While you're out there, I want you to notice a few things.

a. Breath - Should be even, able to hold a conversation. If it's heavy and jagged - walk!

b. Pelvic Floor - Do you feel heaviness, pressure, or leakage - STOP! Gently walk to your starting point. No more running today! Reach back out to your PFPT.

c. Breasts - Is that pre-pregnancy sports bra, or one from during pregnancy doing its job? If not, let's get a new one that fits your post-pregnancy breasts, as they have likely changed and need new support.

d. Feet - Do your feet feel cushioned? Are your arches supported? How about your heels? Any blisters? Feet tend to change size/shape during pregnancy and postpartum. I recommend getting fitted for running shoes at a running specialty shop.

For each of the above, once you have addressed the issue, try another ten-minute run/walk and reassess all of the items. Once you're out there for ten minutes and no issues arise, go to Step 5.

---

[2] Ryan Andrews, MS, MA, RD, RYT, CSCS, "All About Sleep" Precision Nutrition, https://www.precisionnutrition.com/all-about-sleep.

5. COULD I HAVE A CONVERSATION WITH SOMEONE FOR THIS ENTIRE RUN?

YES - Let's look at adding in a second run this week or increasing your total time from your last run by one-to-two minutes.

NO - Slow Down!

One of the quotes I share with my athletes is this:

"If you want to run faster, you need to run farther; if you want to run farther, you need to *slow down!*"

I know it's hard. But you will be optimizing your overall performance in the long run. Okay, so you've found your easy/conversation-pace run, and you're ready to add some mileage. Go to Step 6.

CHECK-IN TIME

6. ARE YOU STILL HAVING FUN?

YES - Great! Go to Step 7.

NO - Circle back to where the fun stopped and reassess.

7. LOOK AT YOUR SCHEDULE BEFORE YOU START MAKING A TRAINING PLAN. CAN YOU FIT RUNNING IN FOR 10-12 MINUTES 2-3 DAYS PER WEEK?

YES - This approach gets you out there building your routine without overloading your schedule with too much time required in one day and minimizes over-stressing your body.

NO - Once a week is all you have time for? That is all you need. Once it becomes a chore, the fun starts to leak out. Keep it fun!

But you may be asking, "But Melissa, when can I start going faster?" Well, remember my quote from above?

I recommend you to be using the easy/conversation pace 80% of the time.[3] The other 20% of the time is where you get to sprint up hills, do a track workout, run with a faster running buddy, or run a race. I know how fun those are, so we want to see them as being allowed.

Below is a sample week for someone training for their first 5k after baby, once in Step 7 for about a month:

Tuesday: Easy/conversation pace run ~2 miles or 15-25 minutes

Thursday: Speed Work ~1-2 miles or 10-20 minutes

Saturday: Easy/conversation pace run ~2-3 miles or 20-40 minutes

Too many times, people run the same hard pace for every run, and that increases your risk for injury, overtraining, fatigue, and burnout! No one has fun running in those scenarios!

Follow these seven steps for an empowered guide to safely return to running while feeling confident with a lowered risk of injury and maintaining your pelvic health.

Lastly, always remember that running should be fun. If it isn't filling your cup, ask yourself why, assess, and just know that it's okay not to run right now.

---

3 Matt Fitzgerald, *80/20 Running: Run Stronger and Race Faster by Training Slower* (Berkley; Illustrated edition, 2014).

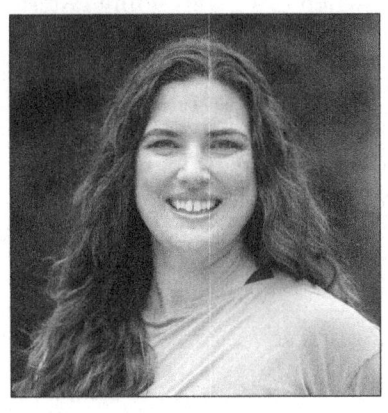

Melissa Szurovy is a runner, lifter, and hockey mom. She loves curling up with a good book on Sunday morning with a hot cup of coffee, although those days are few and far between supporting her kids' extracurricular activities!

She is the owner/head coach of Chesapeake Running Academy and the founder of the StrongMom RunClub. The Chesapeake Running Academy aims to keep running fun for long-term athletic development at any age to live a life full of movement, with education on technique, tactics, and training to excel in sport and reduce the risk of injury while crushing goals along the way.

Melissa is a certified Road Runner Club of America (RRCA) Running Coach, who has been coaching people to run distances from beginner runners to 25k trail runs to full marathons for more than three years.

She holds additional certifications as a National Academy of Sports Medicine certified personal trainer, a Postnatal Fitness Specialist, and a Precision Nutrition Level 1 Coach.

Melissa's devotion to service includes volunteering as a local coach for Girls on the Run, T-ball, the Annapolis Striders juniors running program, and she has co-organized two local youth triathlons and a 5k to fundraise for her neighborhood swim team, is active at her kids' school and serves on her local HOA board.

Melissa is married to her husband Scott, has two very active children, and retired from the United States Navy in 2023.

Find the Chesapeake Running Academy at the links below

www.chesapeakerunningacademy.com

www.facebook.com/chesapeakerunning

www.instagram.com/chesapeakerunning

Join the hundreds of moms in the StrongMom RunClub free community

www.facebook.com/groups/strongmomrunclub

Ready to level up your running with a custom training plan?

Contact Melissa directly melissa@chesapeakerunningacademy.com

CHAPTER 4

42 Days for 42 Years

SIMPLE POSTPARTUM RITUALS FOR LIFELONG HEALTH

Melissa Maxwell, Ayurveda Health Counselor, RYT-500

Before we begin, I want to honor all the mothers, grandmothers, and women healers who passed down these 5,000-year-old traditions—caring for hundreds of generations of mothers and babies before me. Thank you.

MY STORY

I was born to be a supermom. Growing up the oldest of four children, I was changing diapers and warming up bottles before my first day of kindergarten. Taking care of others was imprinted into my identity, and truthfully, I was good at it.

My friends would joke, "I can't believe they let me leave with a baby," when reminiscing about leaving the hospital. I didn't get it. I couldn't wait to get home with my newborn daughter, Mia, so I could transform into a cooking, cleaning, caretaking supermom.

Hard work is in my nature, growing up with two full-time, working parents. My mother had a traditional nine-to-five job, and during most of my childhood, my dad took on side jobs to help pay the bills. We always had everything we needed, but it wasn't without the endless sacrifice of my parents' time, energy, and well-being.

Recently, my mentor asked me, "How was rest modeled for you as a child?"

I had to think hard because I never saw my parents rest unless they were horribly sick. My dad lived off less than six hours of sleep per night for decades—regularly working 18-hour days—and my mom only rested once all four kids were fed, bathed, and tucked in for the night. I rarely saw my mom go for a spa day, and her idea of alone time was grocery shopping. My parents lived to take care of their family, and rest meant someone wasn't doing their part.

I can't even remember my mother resting after the birth of any of my three siblings, but maybe that's because she didn't. Dinners continued to be made, laundry was done, and we never missed a day of school.

So, when it was my turn to experience the postpartum recovery period, I stepped right into my generationally imprinted role of being the caretaker, homemaker, and, ultimately, supermom. I didn't want anyone to think I couldn't handle motherhood, and I made it my goal to squash anyone's thoughts of me needing help.

"Are you sure you'll be okay if I head to a couple of appointments?" Ben, my husband, asked the morning after we brought our daughter, Mia, home. He already knew my answer.

"We'll be great!" I quickly responded. *This is my chance to prove to him that I can handle it all.*

The moment he walked out the door, I jumped up to start cleaning the kitchen. We had been eating takeout since coming home, so I was ready for a home-cooked meal. I whipped up a quick quinoa and chicken stew and then started the laundry - something we had to do daily since Mia was extremely pukey.

What else could I do? I thought, slightly out of breath from walking both flights of stairs in our townhome.

I heard little wails coming from the baby monitor and rushed to the crib. I could feel the stabbing pains of the letdown reflex pierce my chest, my body's response to her cries.

"Let's have lunch together and then go for a walk," I cooed to my cranky, post-nap newborn. We headed downstairs, and every step made my knees ache.

"I'll try to avoid dropping food on you this time," I joked while carefully balancing a bowl of quinoa stew in one hand and carrying Mia in the other. I could sense Mia getting impatient, so I quickly got myself set up to breastfeed on the couch.

After lunch, I strapped Mia into one of our various baby-wearing devices and headed outside.

More stairs, I rolled my eyes as we slowly lumbered down the 15 steps from the front door to the sidewalk. *I'm already exhausted.*

We took a very slow stroll around the block, and I could feel my uterus cramping. Suddenly, a gush of warm liquid soaked the giant menstrual pad I was wearing. *Ugh, I guess it's time to head back.*

Fifteen more steps back into the house, and I could barely catch my breath. My legs were like Jell-O. *Why was that so hard?*

You'd think I'd take the not-so-subtle hints from my body to rest, but I didn't. The next few weeks continued the same, constantly trying to prove I was a supermom.

My body responded with new waves of bleeding. And just when I felt like my uterus was finally healed, I'd stretch my walks 15 minutes longer, and the bleeding would restart.

The Google search bar always knew what I was about to type because of the frequency I searched, "How long does postpartum bleeding last?"

Just after Mia turned four weeks old, we stuffed our truck with baby gear and drove seven hours to the Outer Banks for a week-long family beach vacation.

Nothing about the trip was relaxing. My body ached from sitting in the car, walking on the sand, and sleeping in a crappy bed, and I still bled on and off the entire week.

The following week, I got a text, "Are you ready to start coaching? We need a sub for class this Wednesday." Obviously, I replied with an excited "Yes!"

Though it was fun to do something non-baby-related, standing for hours and moving weights was not what my body craved. I desperately needed rest.

Since my six-week postpartum check-up was only a week away, I decided to hold off on coaching any more classes and instead reached out to my personal training clients, letting them know I was back in business. My schedule filled up quickly.

The next week, I went to see the OB for my appointment.

"Let's check to make sure everything is healing properly. Go ahead and get undressed." He handed me a paper gown, "I'll be back in a moment."

I can't wait to work out again, I thought to myself as I got changed.

"Ready?" my doctor asked through the door.

"Yup!" I replied.

My body felt heavy and cumbersome as I awkwardly scooted to the edge of the examination table.

"A little pressure," he warned and disappeared out of view.

He popped up, "Your cervix is no longer dilated, and your tear healed up well."

"So, I can start working out?" I asked, trying not to sound too eager.

He smiled. "Yes, but go slow, and if you start bleeding again, stop and give me a call."

That same day, I signed up to take a CrossFit-style class. Unfortunately, the dangerous combination of muscle memory and friendly competition led me to push myself harder than I should've; it was a horrible wake-up call.

My body wasn't ready. The 45-minute workout led to four more weeks of bleeding, Googling symptoms, and stress that could have been avoided if I had just listened to my body.

Like many other new mamas, I spent the first six weeks trying to force myself back into normal life. I disregarded proper nourishment and rest as a vital part of the healing process, even when my body was screaming at me to slow down.

Fortunately, three years later, while pregnant with my second baby, I was introduced to the 5,000-year-old healing art called Ayurveda. The word Ayurveda literally translates into "the teachings of life," acknowledging each person as more than a system of organs or diagnosis and rather as a whole being—body, mind, and spirit.

According to the teachings of Ayurveda, the birth experience is not only the birth of a baby but also considered the rebirth of the mother. Meaning that the postpartum period is a reset for the new mother's health. It's a time to rebuild vitality through pure (*sattvic*) foods and restore the balance of the mind and body through daily self-care (*dinacharya*) and rest.

Therefore, the first 42 days postpartum can set the mama up for either a lifetime of imbalances or a lifetime of health.

THE TOOL

This section is not a substitute for professional postpartum care. If you are experiencing pain, bleeding, or signs of postpartum depression, please seek out help from your professional medical care provider.

Throughout the history of childbirth, women have come together to support the new mother during her first six weeks postpartum. In Ayurveda, the new mother is fed healing tonics, warm broths, and nourishing soups; while midwives and doulas wrap the mother's belly, massage her skin with warm oil, and give her sponge baths to prevent getting chilled. Family members visit to clean the mother's home and tend to the baby while she rests.

The first six weeks postpartum is a sacred window of time when the mother is gently nurtured back into a balanced state, rebuilding her reserves after the physical depletion of pregnancy and childbirth while also meeting the energetic demands of breastfeeding and caring for a newborn.

Ayurvedic teachings say that every being is born with a unique constitution (*prakruti*) formed from the three energetic types (*doshas*)— *vata*, *pitta*, and *kapha*. The *doshas* hold the qualities of the five elements:

- *Kapha:* earth and water.
- *Pitta:* fire and a small amount of water.
- *Vata:* air and ether (the space that contains the other four elements).

Every food, experience, and thought has a specific *doshic* energy, and either moves you closer to your original nature (*prakruti*) or creates imbalance in the body or mind (*vikruti*) in the form of discomfort, disorder, or disease.

There is an old Ayurvedic saying, "42 days for 42 years," meaning how a mother is cared for in the first 42 days after birth sets the stage for her next 42 years of health.

The weeks immediately following birth should be dedicated to balancing the overload of *vata dosha* in the mother. As I mentioned, *vata* is made of air and ether and creates excess wind, space, movement, coolness, dryness, and variability in the body. During labor and delivery, *vata dosha* skyrockets due to the intense downward flow of energy (*apana*) created from birth, the physical separation of baby and mama, and the empty space in the mother's body where the baby once was.

I'm grateful to have learned these ancient teachings before birthing my son. From sacred rest and nourishing foods to daily massage, the three postpartum principles I share below are my interpretations of the traditional Ayurvedic rituals used to support the new mama during her transition into motherhood. These principles have been updated for the modern-day mama, who may or may not have family support but desires simple, effective, and easy-to-implement postpartum care options.

POSTPARTUM PRINCIPLE 1: REST

In traditional Ayurveda, mother and baby remain at home, or move into her own mother's home, for the first 42 days, while family members help with household tasks like cooking and cleaning. Today, staying home for 42 days is an unrealistic expectation, and many mamas live hundreds, if not thousands, of miles away from close family.

That said, the modern mama can still implement the principle of rest by staying in bed with the baby as much as possible, minimizing strenuous activity, and avoiding travel beyond the necessary doctor visits for the first 42 days.

Omitting rest during the early postpartum weeks further aggravates *vata dosha*, leading to slower recovery and long-term *vata* imbalances such as poor immune response, weakened digestion, sleep disturbances, and feelings of overwhelm.

Besides good old-fashioned sleep, two simple and highly effective rituals that promote rest and stillness for the overstimulated postpartum body and mind are breath work (*pranayama*) and meditation (*dhyana*).

Pranayama has been used for thousands of years to support the flow of energy (*prana*) in the body. Try this simple *pranayama* practice of presence: Come into stillness; observe each inhale and exhale without judgment; and become aware of where the breath is shallow versus where it is expansive. Notice the prana moving throughout the body—it may feel like warmth, tingling, or lightness.

Complimentary to *pranayama*, meditation is the practice of stilling the mind and body to cultivate relaxation, process thoughts, gain clarity, and relieve chronic stress. There are countless meditation apps available these days, but all you need to meditate is a few minutes to get quiet or still, once or twice a day, while the baby naps or is safely nestled in her crib.

For those who are new to meditation, here are a few tips to get you started:

1. Find a comfortable position, either seated or lying down, where you will not be disturbed. New mamas might find sitting upright in a chair with their back supported to be the most comfortable position for meditation.
2. Close your eyes to remove external distractions and turn your attention inward. Notice your breath, heartbeat, and the conversations occurring in your mind.
3. Welcome a sense of peace and quiet. Allow thoughts to come and go without attachment. Observe feelings that arise in the body. When external distractions pull you away, gently usher your focus back to you.

POSTPARTUM PRINCIPLE 2: FOOD

I recently came across a social media thread asking mothers to share their first meal after childbirth. Their answers included everything from pizza and hamburgers to sushi and even a few cheeky wine emoji comments.

Unfortunately, as delicious as a juicy bacon cheeseburger sounds after 72 hours of labor, heavy, greasy, and excessively salty foods can wreak havoc on a mama's vulnerable postpartum digestion, leading to heartburn, constipation, painful gas, and a build-up of toxins (*ama*).

There are two goals when it comes to postpartum nutrition:

1. Restore vitality (*ojas*) by prioritizing nourishing foods, warming spices, and moisturizing herbal teas to replenish reproductive tissues and support healthy lactation.
2. Rebuild digestive fire (*agni*) by consuming easy-to-digest foods, eating on a regular schedule, and cooking with spices that build and balance *agni*.

In traditional Ayurveda, the new mama is served soft, warm, soupy foods to help rebuild *agni* and ensure that sufficient nutrients are available to nourish all seven tissue layers of the body (*dhatus*), from the first layer of lymph and breast milk (*rasa dhatu*) to the seventh layer of reproductive tissue (*artava dhatu*).

A classic meal for the first few weeks is an easy-to-digest, *vata*-balancing, and *agni*-restoring soupy rice porridge with molasses, spices, and ghee. Since *vata dosha* has a cooling effect on the body after birth, warming spices such as cinnamon, cardamom, ginger, nutmeg, and turmeric are added to the porridge to rekindle digestion and increase warmth. Besides rice porridge, which could be substituted with soupy oatmeal, other foods that help restore vitality to the new mama include soaked dates, warm raw cow's milk, ghee, broths, stewed fruit, and cooked root vegetables.

After two to four weeks, the mama may feel ready to introduce foods like split mung beans and stewed meats, which are both great sources of iron and protein. She should continue to avoid foods that could aggravate *vata dosha*, such as legumes, leftovers, frozen or raw foods, and cruciferous vegetables, while also taking note of any gas, bloating, or constipation. These common digestive symptoms signify that *agni* hasn't been fully restored, and the mama should return to the easier-to-digest food options.

In addition to hydrating with warm or room temperature water (ice cold beverages can further diminish *agni*), the new mama can also sip herbal teas, which help increase warmth and moisture in the body, support digestion, and promote healthy lactation.

Herbs such as shatavari, ashwagandha, and brahmi are highly rejuvenating for postpartum recovery. To ensure proper dosages, the new mama can seek support from a professional herbalist for a postpartum and breastfeeding-safe herbal regimen. In addition, many beneficial teas can be found in standard grocery stores, including ginger for digestion, chamomile for calming, nettle leaf for reducing inflammation, and red raspberry leaf for uterine toning and healthy milk production.

POSTPARTUM PRINCIPLE 3: SELF CARE

For the mama who lives off a mental [or physical] checklist, the first 42 days are the most important time to prioritize intuitive, nurturing self-care rituals. Dedicating this crucial time to caring for herself also sets the new mama up for decades of good health.

With the new demands of feeding, burping, and rocking a newborn, creating a simple daily self-care ritual (*dinacharya*) is an essential practice to ensure the mama is tending to her own needs.

A highly restorative self-care ritual from traditional Ayurveda is a daily warm oil massage (*abhyanga*). Family members or postpartum caretakers provide hour-long *abhyanga* to the new mama every day for the first 30-40 days after birth to help remove excess fluids, relieve aching muscles, and promote contraction of the uterus, returning it to its original size and position.

For modern mamas who don't have the support of close family or a postpartum doula, aiming for two to three shorter, self-performed sessions of *abhyanga* per week with warm sesame oil is sufficient for balancing excess *vata dosha* while also encouraging improvements in circulation, detoxification, and overall stress reduction.

Another postpartum ritual for balancing *vata* is belly wrapping, a technique in which strips of cotton cloth are used to bind the mother's abdomen. This simple postpartum practice is extremely helpful for reducing excess space created after birth, supporting stretched-out core muscles, preventing chronic back pain, and guiding abdominal organs back into their pre-pregnancy position.

You can learn more about abhyanga, belly wrapping, postpartum nutrition, herbal remedies, and rejuvenating self-care rituals in my free downloadable Ayurvedic Postpartum Guide at www.wellbymelissa.com/42-for-42.

These ancient rituals have been practiced for thousands of years because they are simple, effective, and intuitive. Let us follow the wisdom of the generations of women who birthed before us, not only learning to mother our babies but also to mother ourselves.

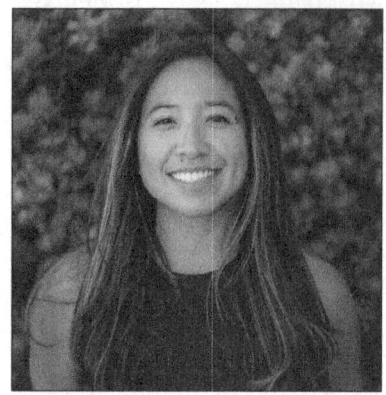

Melissa Maxwell is a certified IIN Holistic Health Coach, Ayurveda Health Counselor, RYT-500, Postpartum Correctional Exercise Specialist, and Reiki Master with over 15 years of experience in women's health, including functional nutrition, strength training, prenatal and postpartum wellness, and trauma-informed yoga. She is the owner of Well by Melissa, a coaching and educational platform for modern and motivated women who desire a more feminine and intuitive approach to wellness.

She believes women can embrace their analytical and ambitious—masculine—qualities while also developing confidence in their femininity through spirituality, mindfulness, and a deeper connection with nature. Melissa has a profound ability to transform ancient wisdom and complex science into simple and effective tools that empower women on their journey to lifelong wellness.

When she's not in the kitchen crafting new recipes, Melissa enjoys doing yoga, snowboarding, reading, traveling, and making new memories with her adventure-loving husband and two adorably energetic children.

Follow Melissa on social media for simple ways to integrate Ayurveda, yoga, and women-specific wellness into everyday life. And visit www.wellbymelissa.com to learn more about coaching opportunities, yoga retreats, virtual and in-person workshops, and all other Well by Melissa offerings.

Melissa Maxwell

Email: hello@wellbymelissa.com

Website: https://www.wellbymelissa.com

Instagram: https://www.instagram.com/wellbymelissa/

Facebook: https://www.facebook.com/wellbymelissa/

CHAPTER 5

What to Do When the Cat in the Hat is You

FOLLOWING YOUR FUN INTO A LIFE YOU LOVE

Robin Lee Arnesen, Pilates Teacher

MY STORY

Quieting Outside Energy, Learning About Yourself, and Leaning Into the Life You Love.

"Yes. It is real," I said, getting annoyed at my new Facebook marketplace BFF, who I was meeting for the first time in a well-lit parking lot.

"Like even if I bothered to try and sell a fake bag, I'm selling this real Chanel for cheaper than a decent fake," I continued.

"Trust me, I'm not the kind of person to sew a fake bag, and not because I'm super honest, because as much as I work out and run around, I'm really kind of lazy about other things," my mouth said as it handed over complete control to my ADHD.

"It's actually a funny story about how I got this bag! I was working for Bayer, you know, like Asprin, and there was this place way north of Baltimore, and my friend called me and was like…" I rambled.

"Yeah, okay, here's $500.00," my Facebook marketplace soul mate said to me, trying to get out of the well-lit parking lot and away from me as fast as she could.

I'll mention my ADHD again now.

"Sweet! I've got more. Message me if you're interested. Oh! I'm late for my apprenticeship! Bye!"

In my mind, she muttered something like, "Later, Johnny Tremain." After all, she was clever enough to sniff out and score a deal on a real Chanel bag. She seemed down for some 8th-grade literature humor.

In reality, I'm sure she assumed "apprenticeship" was code for a different kind of deal. It wasn't. I was selling bags in the parking lot of a gym on the daily to pay for Pilates teacher training.

And like a flash of silver, I was off to the studio!

This became my pattern for a while—selling my things in a parking lot and turning the cash around to pay for Pilates teacher training. Wow. O'Henry really was on to something with that Gift of the Magi stuff.

How did I get here—selling purses out of my car in a gym parking lot?

As a young adult and as a wife, before I became a mother, I worked as a pharmaceutical sales rep. I did really well when I wasn't playing hooky buying Chanel bags. I did well; ADHD brains are motivated by urgency and competition. Still, I woke up each day riddled with anxiety and guilt. But whatever, I could push through till we could comfortably live on one income.

It was just a placeholder, a pit stop on the way to Stay-at-Home-Mom-Land. The goal was always to be a Stay-at-Home-Mom. In some toxic friend groups, it felt like a race to get there, like some sub-strain of Keeping Up with the Joneses, which felt a lot like Jonestown to me. As someone motivated by competition, I arrived quickly at Stay-at-Home-Mom-Land, and it was "auf Wiedersehen pharma!" Finally! I could just stay at home.

Then, I didn't work for 12 years. I do not mean to say, "I didn't work outside the home." I did not work. Terrible stay-at-home mom and a bad wife.

"Please, just leave me alone and let me get this done!" I said through professionally whitened gritted teeth while I stuck two cloves in a marshmallow and put it on a toothpick with tissue around it.

I did this 30 times over as I volunteered to bring the pre-school Halloween snack. This is what proves I'm a good mom. I have to do it, and I will; it will look great in the end, but it will be ugly getting there. Yes, I'm still talking about a marshmallow ghost. This rage is not Halloween project-specific. It could've been any cutesy craft on any given half-day of school holiday.

Should I be making marshmallow ghosts that invoke rage aimed at the children I'm making them for? Everyone else seems to think so, and everyone else seems to enjoy it. What is this?

I did not work at all in any way inside the home. It definitely did not work for me. I'll have the self-loathing with extra guilt, please.

I appeared to be a good stay-at-home mom thanks to ADHD masking and motivational deadlines. A husband returning from work or friends coming over for an easy gourmet dinner would snap me into action enough to make everything look right. When I was alone with my kids and able to take the mask off, I was a yelling mom—scarier and way more confusing and let's face it, memorable, than a masking mom or a marshmallow ghost.

I was surrounded by so many of the things I didn't know I didn't need. For 36 years, outside energy set my goals: Stay-at-home mom life, car, house, husband, kids, and from there, more accumulation.

It was not what I wanted, but I didn't know it. As I did in my drug rep career, I felt anxious and guilty all the time. *How can anyone not be happy with all this? It's what everyone wants.*

It's no one's fault, but like all the Disney movies, growing up ended with a wedding. It was not what I wanted.

People in my life knew I was unhappy with my label as mom and wife, but they couldn't understand why.

Outside energy source: "You won't be driving that nice car anymore."

Outside energy source: "Every woman in your situation loses the fancy SUV."

Outside energy source: "You can't leave and keep driving that car."

Am I crazy? Is this car the key to my happiness?

Invoking a great Carrie Bradshaw pun, I must say.

I lost the trust I had in others' opinions, even those closest to me. I needed self-reliance. I re-read my journals like movie scenes. Yeah, I don't think missing the car is worth staying.

So, I blew it up. I left. I took my kids with me. They are awesome. I quit the rest of it. It was active. I did things I knew the life I had would never recover from. I faced everything I thought I feared most.

In a series of events, I took the mask off forever and knew I could never wear it again. I threw the secure future away with it.

I was stripped of my wife title, and the judges were looking at my mom crown with some major side-eye. I didn't care. I wanted to know who I was. I spent the money I got in the divorce to pay for the divorce. I knew that would happen and just thought about it like Scarlett O'Hara and continued to think about it tomorrow. So, there I was.

I always journaled for catharsis. But I was lost. I knew what I did not want anymore. I knew that I hadn't felt quite like myself in a long time.

I began my Odyssey.

I went down a rabbit hole via my journals to educate myself about myself. The act of journal writing is cathartic and cleansing, but it also contains invaluable information for you as the main character.

I read the stories about myself written by myself, and I found patterns.

I continued to read my journals like a book. Entries span genres, and whether or not you love or hate the main character, they give great insights into her mind and into her world.

Cute! At 16, her dad gave her a Pilates DVD to keep her strong and injury-free for a long lacrosse career.

Wow! She's super happy! She did a fitness modeling gig at a Pilates studio and had so much fun.

Oh, this one's sad. She's upset because she wanted to try Pilates teacher training and she can't because she doesn't have the time. She is really upset.

Reading my journals, seeing my pictures, and listening to myself gave me the confidence to know that Pilates is what I wanted to build my life around.

I learned from scribbled notes that when I put energy into Pilates, I got energy back. I realized none of my journal entries described the joy in a bag; I never deliberately captured a picture of Prada like I do my kids and dogs.

"I am literally a bag lady." I wrote in cursive in my journal, Carrie again, the Sex and the City episode when Carrie realizes she spent all her money on shoes and has nowhere to live.

I had bags and shoes I didn't want and a career I did want. Okay, this makes sense to my ADHD brain. I can make this work. I will sell my stuff and take the apprenticeship.

Then, snapping back into Scarlet O'Hara recovery mode, I gathered up my high-end bags and shoes and, for the first time, deliberately took pictures of all my stuff, got a snack, and listed it all on the Facebook marketplace. If I could sew, I totally would have ripped down the drapes.

So here I was, Robin Lee Arnesen, privileged with the finest education money can buy, selling luxury items in the parking lot of a gym to pay for my classical Pilates apprenticeship.

Seriously, I have a very expensive Irish Literature degree, and I have tied sheets together and shimmed out a window. If you learn nothing from me, please take away that boarding school only begets the bad behavior that gets one sent away to boarding school.

Red Manolo Blahnik Mary Janes parlayed into a day of learning short spine massage. Makes good business sense, too. For months, I brokered these deals, and after many hours of training, I am a Pilates teacher, a label I love.

Eventually, all the stuff was gone, and with it, the noise. I'm left simply with a life I love. I support myself and my family with a beautiful career, helping humans feel safe, strong, and powerful in their bodies. Teaching humans to move their bodies with efficiency, purpose, and freedom has allowed me to move through life with efficiency, purpose, and freedom. I am a Pilates teacher—a good Pilates teacher, a happy Pilates teacher. It's a label I like. It's a lifestyle that made sense and allowed me to make peace with other labels like mom. Wife? Not yet. I can't say I never yelled again, but I saved us from a life with a yelling mom.

My oldest said to me: "I like that you never say 'I have to work,' you just say what you're going to do. And you always come and go happy."

"I am going to train Jules."

"Today, I will teach Anita to do a push-up."

"I'll help Scott prepare for his golf tournament."

"I will laugh with Nancy as we stretch and strengthen."

"I will help Ester and Minson become Pilates teachers themselves."

We will move with efficiency, purpose, and freedom.

THE TOOL

SIMPLIFY: SPIRAL IN AND SPIRAL OUT.

Without the pressure of numbers, calendars, schedules, etc., allow time (whenever you can allow time) for absolutely zero stimuli. No music, no journal prompts, no noise, no guides, and as little outside energy as possible.

When you add back in, where do your instincts take you? When I am ready to reconnect, I add back movement, music, and usually coffee. I write this down and look for patterns of consistency. Movement, music, coffee…

And when I do invite living, breathing outside energy in, I usually reconnect with my children and my dog

ADHD paralysis will put me here involuntarily. Everything will just stop, and I, to use the technical term, zone out. This typically happens when tasked with something my brain is just not going to want to do. I taught myself to use the time.

Okay, like I would rather die than fold laundry. So, I'm going to sit here, and someone will probably someday just do it for me because somebody always helps that girl.

The people say to meditate, so if my brain will not let me move to be productive, I'm calling this meditation and getting credit for it.

Okay, so it doesn't look like this laundry is going to Fantasia-style fold itself. Okay. Fine. But first, I'm putting on music, a spine stretch forward, and getting a coffee.

Whether it's meditation or ADHD paralysis, there is truth in your reconnect. Notice what you gravitate back to.

SELL YOURSELF YOURSELF. USE YOUR SOCIAL MEDIA TO FALL IN LOVE WITH YOUR LIFE.

Hi. I am Robin, and I love social media. Hi Robin.

Whether it's evil or not, it's here to stay and a vital part of a career in fitness. I use it to grow my business, and I use it to grow my love for the life I live.

Similar to my career as a punk girl, my career as a photographer is mostly in my imagination. But I love to sing and pogo dance, and I love taking pictures. Capturing the minutia of my days and finding small moments of beauty, humor, and vulnerability keeps me curious, observant, and present. Small moments—my dog walking, the coat check at The Anthem D.C., a Pilates exercise, a Pilates exercise fail, and my kid's face in the window of the bus—have all helped me to love the human experience. I notice what is important enough for me to notice. Unsure that I will get to experience being a human again, I like to record the moments now. Throw in that this child of the 90s can add music and create my own little music video, and did I mention that I love social media? It's my modern-day journal.

If I come off as self-absorbed, it's because I am. Anyway, unless I'm specifically looking for something like a classical Pilates studio to recommend to friends in their area, I really only look at my own social media. Creating stories about the happiest, most interesting, and quirkiest parts of my life allows me to actively show gratitude for it. I post it, yes, because maybe it brings amusement to another human, and if not, they can keep scrolling. But I've learned to let go of likes. I rewatch and admire that I'm beautiful, strong, and funny. Without outside energy telling me so, I know this.

What are you feeding yourself?

I found a library card from 2nd grade. In 1987, I checked out *Amelia Bedelia*. I grew up to be a quirky but loveable terrible housekeeper.

Revisit the outside energies that, for better or worse, shaped your life. I watched *Friends* and *Seinfeld* every Thursday. I thought I was Rachel all along; turns out I'm Phoebe and Elaine.

My favorite movie as a kid was *What Away to Go*, starring Shirley Maclain as a woman just looking for a simple life.

I have read *Fight Club* more than any other book.

When my children were babies, I read them Yeats.

And I am the girl in every song.

What makes you love and relate to a character? What outside energy do you

Free Writing: I majored in Irish Literature, and while I don't use it a lot, I still enjoy it past my formal education. I concentrated on my favorite poet, W.B. Yeats. I learned free writing from Yeats, a style of journaling. You ask a question and just write without conscious thought. Read your answers like you're reading a book. Study yourself, observe, learn, apply. Make it raw, simple, and real.

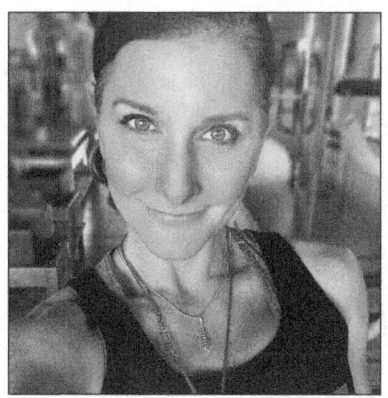

Robin Lee Arnesen works as a Pilates teacher at Chesapeake Pilates Center in Annapolis, Maryland. Robin completed her first Pilates Certification in Annapolis in 2017. In 2022, Robin graduated from Alycea Ungaro's Real Pilates Teacher Training in New York, New York.

Robin also works as a real estate agent in Maryland for Keller Williams.

Robin attended Bucknell University in Lewisburg, Pennsylvania, where she majored in Irish Literature and played lacrosse. She still coaches lacrosse and studies Irish Literature.

Robin lives on Maryland's Eastern Shore with her children Millz, Will, and their German Shepherd, Chuck. They spend their free time in nature, camping, and by the water.

Robinleepilates@gmail.com

@chesapeakepilatescenter

@shapeshifterrla

CHAPTER 6

The Myth of the Good Mother

HOW TO ASK FOR HELP

Maria Winters, LCPC, NCC

MY STORY

Snowmaggedon! That's what they called it. When my water broke at 6 am, I immediately called my OB-GYN. Her advice was clear: "Don't come here. Don't risk getting stranded. Go to a closer hospital." Panic set in. *I am doomed!*

It was February 2010 in Maryland, and the snowfall was at levels no one expected. We were hit with about 50 inches of snow after back-to-back blizzards. Flights were canceled, roofs collapsed, neighborhoods were without power, schools shut down, and motorists were stranded. The city struggled to keep up; there was simply too much snow and nowhere to pile it all.

During one of the blizzards, our house lost both power and water, just two weeks away from my due date. My husband opted to book a nearby hotel for us. We packed some essentials, including snacks and refrigerated food, to save them from our powerless home. If there's one thing I learned throughout my pregnancy, it's the importance of always having snacks available to combat hunger pangs.

Together with my husband, mother, and our dog, we relocated to the hotel, my heavily pregnant belly in tow. We checked in and decided to grab something to eat at the hotel's restaurant. As soon as we sat down, the waitress said, "Due to the storms, we haven't received food deliveries for days, so I'm sorry to inform you that half the items on the menu aren't available." Thankfully, our stash of snacks and provisions came to the rescue.

I remember that mixed feeling of "nervcited"—nervous yet excited, knowing my baby could come any minute. Then came the next morning when we discovered a plow truck that got stuck sideways at the entrance of the hotel, blocking all access to the road. This meant that, if labor came, our only option would be to walk about four blocks, in the snow, to the main road and hope for a taxi or ambulance to reach us. There was not much excitement anymore, only pure nervousness. *Breathe in, breathe out. Am I doomed?*

The truck was eventually removed, power returned to our house, and I didn't go into labor. So, we returned home. *Ah, home sweet home.* Things started feeling a bit normal until another blizzard struck. The Weather Channel was warning us of record accumulations, advising everyone to stay home. And then, my water broke. I contacted my OB-GYN, who said: "Don't come here. Don't risk getting stranded. Go to a closer hospital."

Back then, I lived 17 miles from the hospital where I intended to give birth and where my OB-GYN practiced. Another hospital, just four miles from our house, recently opened its labor and delivery unit. Amidst the snowstorm, the closer hospital became the only choice.

The city looked like a scene from a post-apocalyptic movie. It was silent with cars abandoned, emergency lights flashing, roads blocked, and very few vehicles in front of us, slipping and skidding. I couldn't help to think, *I'm going to be one of those women who gives birth in a car!*

Upon our arrival at the hospital, we learned there was no staff relief for a few days due to the storms. A small team of nurses and physicians rotated duties, attempting to grab brief naps between tasks. The first nurse we met told us she had been on shift for over 20 hours. I'm talking exhausted, drained, and significantly overworked medical staff, all stretched very thin. *I am so doomed!*

After 13 hours of IV medication for labor induction, contractions, nurses coming in to discuss my lack of dilation, strained communication between my mom and husband due to her limited English and his limited Spanish, and more contractions, the decision for a C-section was made at 8:30 p.m. A beautiful baby girl entered the world—my beautiful baby girl. As our eyes met, I started sobbing. She was finally here; she was okay. It was all worth it.

I was rolled to a recovery room. I was shaking uncontrollably, so much I couldn't speak—a probable effect of the anesthesia. I felt exhausted, physically and emotionally. I felt fragile and depleted. I wanted to rest. I needed a hug.

Moments later, a nurse came in with my baby. "Hello, momma, let's start breastfeeding." The nurse emphasized the benefits of the colostrum. I was now a mother, entrusted with the sole ability to nourish my child. Exhausted as I was, the weight of motherhood settled in. I still needed a hug.

I returned home, wrapped in the excitement of having my first kid. My mom and husband were a big help for several weeks, but my mom eventually went back home overseas, and my husband went back to work. Reality set in when I found myself alone at home, responsible for a tiny human who needed all my attention. That's when the real storm hit. Forget about the snowmageddon I had just experienced; I was about to weather an emotional storm.

I was raised in a Latin family where everyone was involved in each other's lives, where we saw each other often and lent a hand whenever a family member needed support. I grew up surrounded by a strong tribe, a village. But I didn't have a village here. I was alone and lonely. Those first months of motherhood were proof to me that this journey is not meant to be tackled alone. Not having a village here hurt very much.

I also found myself swept up in a storm of societal and self-imposed expectations and impossibly high standards. I wanted to be a super mom, one that others would admire and feel proud of, one that gave it all for her child, one that did everything to secure a safe and happy childhood.

The pressure started to mount to breastfeed and never use formula, pump milk in between, complete other tasks while the baby napped, keep the house clean, engage the baby's curiosity, and do the laundry. The demands of motherhood were exceeding my ability to manage it all, stretching beyond what I could offer at that moment. I started experiencing mental fatigue; I was short-tempered, and I was feeling emotionally drained and disconnected. I felt guilty for not enjoying every second of it, for not being the mother who took her baby on long stroller walks or laid on the floor for hours to stimulate her. I felt far from well put together or pretty. I also began grieving the loss of my independence, autonomy, sleep, hobbies, dreams, and my pre-pregnancy body.

As a mental health therapist, I've long understood the power of conversation in relieving pressure and sparking insight. Talking has often been my go-to tool and makes me feel better when done with the right people. So, I began reaching out and expressing my feelings and thoughts with friends, family, a therapist, and fellow moms, realizing that I wasn't navigating this journey alone.

Upon opening up about my own struggles, I discovered more women began sharing their struggles. Even those that looked like they had it all under control. It was life-changing for me to find other women with whom I could talk about the sucky parts of motherhood without being judged or my struggles being minimized.

During my many conversations, it became evident that feelings of overwhelm, disconnection, frustration, sadness, isolation, thoughts of suicide, burnout, resentment, and fatigue were more common than I thought. Women shared things like, "I feel like I have too much on my plate and feel constantly pulled from different angles," "I have moments where I wish I could run away," or "I have moments where I feel extreme exhaustion, and all I need is some sleep." Some disliked their lives even when they loved their child with all their heart. Many of us talked about the pressure we felt to do it all or most of it, to do it well, and to have a positive attitude while doing it. Many were reluctant to share their feelings because a baby is expected to bring happiness and joy.

The daily demands of caregiving, coupled with feeling ineffective, the pressure to become better at what I was doing, feelings of disconnection from myself, and persistent doubts about my parenting abilities, were a lot to carry. And here is the thing: all of these can contribute to increased risk for depression, anxiety, hopelessness, and helplessness.

For me, for many years, being a good mother meant preparing home-cooked meals, volunteering at my kids' school, helping with every homework assignment, shielding them from all harm, understanding their needs and satisfying those needs, fostering independence, being emotionally available all the time, remaining calm during challenges, having fun plans for every weekend, keep our house well-decorated and clean, laughing together frequently, playing board games as a family after dinner, and ensuring they didn't make wrong decisions, among many other ideals. I used to compare myself to other moms.

This notion of being the perfect mom was killing me softly. It was making it hard to breathe. It brought out this inner critic I never heard so loud before. This perfect mom thing was not only unrealistic, but it was also making me neglect myself. I realized I was not going to make it by giving it all because If I gave all of myself, then what would be left?

There came a day when I figured out that being a good mom didn't mean sacrificing every bit of myself. It sounds obvious now, but I understood I wouldn't physically be able to attend to my child's every need every moment of the day. I had to let go of preconceived perceptions and beliefs of what motherhood should look like. I knew I needed to find my unique way to motherhood, one that worked for me and my children and one based on our current needs, values, personality types, and the tools I had available. I started giving myself permission not to be a good or bad mother but a real one.

I know now that I can't do it all or be available for my family all the time and that I cannot be everything to my children. I learned I couldn't be much help to anyone if I didn't put my mental and emotional health first.

Being a good mother doesn't mean I have to forget about my plans, desires, goals, dreams, or aspirations. I ditched the comparison, and I made peace with the mother I am. My way of mothering is based on what I have and what I know, and it's an awesome and unique way. *I am NOT doomed at all. I have been blessed, and I am a beautiful work in progress.* It wasn't about surviving anymore; it was about thriving.

Please don't think I've mastered motherhood. I haven't. Motherhood is a continual practice. Some days are great, some days are good, and some days are not that good. But I go through my days without trying to fit into anybody else's standards. I will die one day like everyone else and will think of my motherhood journey with Frank Sinatra in mind, singing:

"Yes, there were times I'm sure you knew,

When I bit off more than I could chew

But through it all, when there was doubt

I ate it up and spit it out

I faced it all and I stood tall and **did it my way**."

I want to share with you, beautiful woman, that you are not a bad mother if motherhood feels hard. You're not a bad mother if you miss having your independence, if sitting on the floor playing with the kids isn't your thing, if you've got dreams for when they're off to college, if alone time brings you joy, if you need those long breaks, and if you've got plans that don't scream 'Mom.'

I also want to tell you that the needs of your kids are very important, but so are yours. You don't have to do it all. What you choose to do doesn't have to be well done all the time. It's okay if there are many things that you do half-ass. Motherhood is not a synonym for suffering.

I invite you to join me in exploring the transformative potential of two simple yet profound actions for our wellbeing. These are powerful yet often overlooked aspects that can pave the way to a more fulfilling and balanced journey as mothers.

THE TOOL

There were two things that the moms I talked to (including myself) were not doing despite having all the evidence that showed how important it was to do it.

- Asking for help
- Allowing others to help and accepting help

This might sound obvious or simple, but it's a game-changer tool available to all and not well used.

I needed help, and a lot of it. However, the expectation to do it all made me feel like I couldn't reach out for help even when I really needed it. There I was with dark circles under my eyes, experiencing frequent irritable and grumpy moods, without showering, and having crying spells but not asking for help.

Asking for help has always been tough for me. My inner critic usually tells me I should be able to do it on my own. I was waiting for my husband and other people around me to figure out what I needed. But here's the thing: no one can read your mind, so I had to internalize that it's not other people's job to know what we need. We can and need to ask for what we need.

Many women, including myself, come from a society that has historically placed on women the task of raising a family. We're the ones who should care for our kids. So, what happens is that a lot of women hold this idea as they become mothers and then feel ashamed when they don't quite match up to those expectations. We try to do it all on our own, and reaching out for help can bring feelings of guilt and unworthiness. In my case, I felt like asking for help meant that I wasn't able to do the simple things I was meant to do as a mother.

It's so important to find people who can help—your tribe! These people can be your partner, neighbors, old friends, new friends, family members, other moms, professionals, a company you hire, or a service provider you outsource to. Find people who can help you with different things. It doesn't matter where you find help as long as you have it. Motherhood can feel so much easier with help.

I want to share with you a few tips on how to ask for help.

I invite you to start by asking yourself: What do I need right now? **Identify the areas where you could have assistance**. It might be household chores, childcare, emotional support, or personal time. Once you have an idea of what you need, approach the person and **communicate it openly**. Express your needs directly and with clarity.

Be specific about what kind of help you need. Specific requests are easier for others to understand and fulfill.

Set realistic expectations: Understand that not everyone can assist in the same way or at the same time. Be open to various forms of support.

Practice self-compassion and grace: Remember, asking for help doesn't make you weak. It's a sign of strength, resourcefulness, and self-awareness. No need to be hard on yourself or measure your effectiveness as a mother based on how much you do all by yourself.

Accept help, even if it doesn't match your exact needs or even when you know others might not do the task as well as you would. Be as flexible as possible. Say yes to help.

Use support services: Consider professional services like babysitting, housekeeping, grocery delivery, a mom's helper, or therapy if available and within your means.

Express gratitude: Appreciate the help you receive. Expressing gratitude encourages continued support and strengthens your relationships.

Need some examples of how to ask for help? Here are a few ideas:

"Hey, I'm feeling overwhelmed with chores this week. Could you help with grocery shopping, bringing meals, or laundry?"

"I need a break and time for myself. Would you mind watching the baby for a couple of hours?"

"I've been feeling stressed lately. Can we schedule a time to talk? Your perspective could help."

"Could you run some errands for me?"

"I'm feeling a bit overwhelmed. Could you help me organize/clean the house?"

"I'm feeling exhausted. Can we discuss how we can share household duties more evenly?"

"I have a lot on my plate right now. Can we explore the option of hiring help a few times a week and/or outsourcing some tasks?"

"I could use some help, but I'm not sure exactly what. Can we brainstorm some ways you might be able to assist?"

Remember, everyone needs a little support sometimes, especially mothers. There's one thing I wish I could tell every tired mother out there, and that is: **It's okay to ask for help**.

Today, my girls are 9 and 14. My unique approach to motherhood is going well. I am emotionally present for my girls but also for myself. I make a lot of mistakes. I own up to them and apologize. My big aim? Showing my girls that taking care of yourself comes first, so we break the habit of putting ourselves last. I model for them that setting limits for ourselves and protecting our energy doesn't mean we are selfish. We frequently talk about the importance of asking for help and how it positively impacts our overall well-being.

MENTAL HEALTH RESOURCES:

You can dial 988 from anywhere in the United States for mental health-related situations that require immediate assistance.

Postpartum Support International: 1-800-944-4773

National Maternal Mental Health Hotline: 1-833-9-HELP4MOMS (1-833-943-5746) call or text

National Suicide Prevention Hotline: 1-800-273-8255

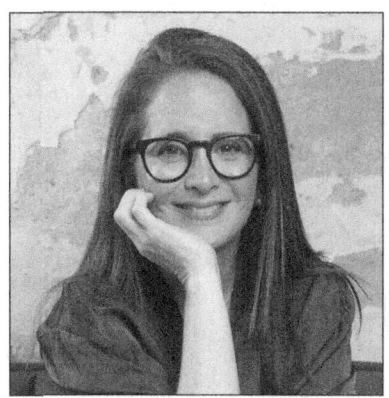

Maria Winters is a licensed mental health therapist and a National Certified Counselor. She is the owner of The Coaching Therapist, LLC, a practice dedicated to providing workshops on mental health related topics. For the past 12 years, Maria has been conducting safety risk evaluations for patients of all ages in a local emergency room. She also offers emotional support groups for women. Maria has more than 18 years of experience providing support to adults and adolescents in a variety of settings including community clinics, foster care, juvenile detention, psychiatric day hospital, and private practice. She has been teaching Psychology at a local community college for over ten years. Maria was born and raised in Venezuela and moved to the United States in the year 2000. She completed her bachelor's degree in psychology at Northeastern University in Boston, Massachusetts, and a master's degree in counseling psychology at Argosy University in Washington, DC. She is a wife and mother of 2 girls and a Bernedoodle, Ringo. Maria is a trained Flamenco dancer and loves dancing on stage. However, any kind of dancing makes her very happy. She is fully bilingual in English and Spanish. Maria is on a mission to help others learn tools to cultivate their mental health. She offers a lighthearted take on emotional health and sees the importance of opening and normalizing these conversations. People appreciate her energetic personality and her use of humor. Maria strives to make emotional wellness something that everyone appreciates and prioritizes. Check out Maria's upcoming workshops at www.thecoachingtherapist.com. Also, go take a listen to her podcast Wellness Rebranded, where she gets together with a dietitian and a personal trainer to promote genuine wellness from three different healing perspectives.

Connect with Maria:
Website: https://thecoachingtherapist.com/
Instagram: @coaching_therapist
Facebook: MWcoachingtherapy
LinkedIn: https://www.linkedin.com/in/maria-winters-98183766
Podcast: Wellness Rebranded

CHAPTER 7

Think Outside the Box

FIVE CREATIVE WAYS TO GET YOUR SEXY BACK

Julie Blamphin, Speaker, Founder of Stretch Your Spirit

DISCLAIMER

You've just read my subtitle that seems to indicate you've "lost your sexy" and are looking for ways to get it back. Perhaps this hasn't happened (yet). But I'm sorry to say that it may be at some point in the future. In spite of that, it doesn't mean you're powerless! We women are prone to feeling disconnected from our sacred feminine energy, but that doesn't mean something is wrong. It means we're all in this together, sister. We're human. We're women. So, let's think outside the box and get creative.

This chapter is personal. I hope you feel as moved while reading it as I felt while writing it.

MY STORY

I was fifty-one years old when I learned that pain during sex isn't normal. It's common, but that doesn't mean it's normal. This condition, called dyspareunia, occurs because of physical and/or emotional reasons and presents itself as chronic pain that occurs before, during, and/or after insertion of a tampon, finger, penis, toy, etc. This was my reality for almost thirty years, and I had no idea it was even a thing.

Here's my theory on how this began and unfortunately continues, although thankfully not as often. And now I know what to do about it.

I was a gymnast in my childhood and teenage years. Gymnastics practice was literally on my daily docket from age six to sixteen. That sport packed a power in my body that I still feel today. It wasn't just the drills, tumbling, and routines but also the intensity to stay focused on perfection.

I also played soccer, ran the 100m hurdles in track, and was on the cheerleading squad. Then, in college, I was a swimmer, diver, weight lifter, and kickboxer. Through it all, I skied as often as possible—water and snow. To say my body was in constant *beast mode* is an understatement.

I noticed the pain in my 20s. Figuring it was a trigger from that time in the woods when _____ pinned my arms down and assaulted me, I've dealt with it the best I know how. In my 30s, I experienced an egg donation process (that failed), further disconnecting me from my sexual energy. The pain persisted. Anxiety then became my copilot, and low libido my middle name. And in my 40s, I experienced a total loss of hearing in my right ear. One evening in May of 2014, as I was crumpled on the floor, spinning wildly from vertigo (that's never fully gone away), I assumed this was my challenge of a lifetime. Actually, it was an amazing opportunity.

It was the impetus behind the next ten years of my research and work. What I realize now is that while trying to solve one mystery, I solved another. As I was diving into the details of the inner ear, balance, and how to manage my new reality, I uncovered clues that were tied to my low libido and pain. That's when I started to think outside the box about my issues. Check this out.

The deep core of the body includes sixteen muscles and fascia at the base of the torso, called the pelvic floor. This area provides support for our internal organs and helps us with balance, bathroom habits, and sexual activity. As it turns out, my pelvic floor muscles have been clenching way too much and way too often ever since I was a child. No wonder I've been feeling pain!

Since these discoveries, I've developed a freedom in my body that's changed my life, and not just my sex life. Through yoga, chakra work, and fascia release, I manage my symptoms of imbalance, clenching, pain, and low libido. Now, I share this with as many women who'll listen.

FUEL TO THE FIRE

In 2022, I was the featured speaker at a women's wellness event. Afterward, a few women lined up to chat with me. Laura was the first.

"My baby is now thirteen years old, and I haven't had sex since before she was born."

She laughed awkwardly.

"And really have no desire to ever again."

Earlier, I asked the women to share with each other how they felt about their sexuality. I noticed Laura was joking around, and a few others were too.

"What sexuality?"

"My sex life is nonexistent."

"That ship has *sailed*, honey!"

They were all on the same page, and each comment was laced with sarcasm and bitterness.

Relatable? Maybe, maybe not. No wrong answers here.

To be frank, their comments weren't surprising. I've worked with hundreds of women since launching Stretch Your Spirit in 2009. From sacred circles at my retreats to business networking events to email questionnaires, I've gained a perspective that fuels the fire behind my work. Yes, my research concluded that general concerns include core strength, insomnia, pain, and leakage, but it seems the top commonality among women is low sex drive.

> *"I don't think you realize how helpful it was for me to come see you postpartum, Julie. You totally helped me get my head right! Not just being a mom, the maker of milk, and the vessel that provides for this baby, but me. I'm still a sexual being. I want to feel good, and you helped me tap into that. I'm worth it! I deserve to feel sexy and sexual."*
>
> ~ Tara De Leon, lead author, *Hot Mess to Hot Mom*

IN REAL LIFE

Low sex drive (or loss of libido) presents itself with **symptoms** such as:

- having no interest in sex or masturbation;
- rarely or never thinking of sex; or
- being unhappy with your low desire for sexual activity or thoughts of sex.

The **causes** of low sex drive are too many to count. Here's a list, and there's undoubtedly more.

- Vaginal dryness
- Painful sex
- Difficulty reaching orgasm
- Hormonal changes
- Pregnancy
- Breastfeeding
- Anxiety/Depression
- Poor body image
- Operations/Procedures
- Exhaustion/Overwhelm
- Relationship difficulties
- History of unwanted sexual contact
- Medication
- Menopause
- Stress
- Dysfunction/Disease
- Mind/Body disconnection[1]

Let's explore that last one on the list: Mind/Body disconnection. Being that the definition of *yoga* is basically a mind/body connection, please keep your hopes up. I got you! Rest assured, feeling disconnected doesn't mean you can't reconnect.

The modern word *yoga* comes from the ancient word yug. Sounds like yoke, yes. Like an egg yoke, yoga binds. It's your connection between mind, body, and spirit. And this connection is a practice.

Pro Tip: Instead of focusing on performance: penetration, positions, toys, and masturbation, let's focus on practice: gentle movement, breathing, mindset, and meditation. Yesss—this is where it gets good.

THE TOOL

PRACTICE

Every day, in some way, practice in real life! I'm not (directly) suggesting you masturbate on the family room floor, but hey, you do you. Sounds like a perfect plan to me.

Simply think outside the box and be creative. Let your practice be your playground, and have fun with it! Remember: sexuality is your energy of creation and creativity. This section contains lots of ideas.

Pro Tip: Pick one you love and practice it as often as possible.

FIVE CREATIVE WAYS TO GET YOUR SEXY BACK

1. MANTRA

A mantra (or affirmation) is a sound, word, or phrase that, when repeated, can provide positive transformation. This is the most powerful way to manifest your intentions. Give your mind something to do with a mantra.

Pro Tip: Please keep it positive and present tense.

A few examples:

I am practicing.

I feel creative and joyful.

I am sexy and fabulous.

Iris Krasnow, author of *Sex After...Women Share How Intimacy Changes As Life Changes* tells us this: "If we can adapt our minds to our changing bodies, anything is possible in sexuality."[2]

Remember I said a mantra can be a sound? Here's my absolute favorite: a sigh.

Do you ever sigh and those around you ask, "What's wrong?"

Yep. I often sigh when times get tough—when I'm frustrated, exasperated, or pissed. I also sigh when I'm feeling motivated, organized, and pleased. I sigh a *lot*. One could say I'm obsessed with the sigh. It just feels good.

A sigh somehow signals negativity, but it totally gets a bad rap. In actuality, it's a positive practice! Here's why. A sigh creates a pause, like a reboot or calibration technique. It's the quickest way to intentionally calm the body and mind. Bonus: It works every time.

"A sigh is a psychophysiological disruptor," says Dr. Patricia Gerbarg, a psychiatrist, co-author of *The Healing Power of the Breath*, and co-founder of the Breath-Body-Mind Foundation, which teaches breathwork to survivors of disaster. "Signals from the respiratory system have top priority over pretty much any other signal from the body, especially when there's a sudden change. So when you change your pattern of breathing, you suddenly change all of the signaling up to the brain."[3]

Think about it. You're having a moment. Maybe you're exhausted, overwhelmed, feeling impatient, and burnt out. Why *wouldn't* you sigh?

Here we go. Take a big breath in through your nose.

Now open your mouth and exhale with a sigh, "Ahhhh..."

Take another breath in.

Again, exhale with a long sigh.

One more big breath in!

Exhale with a long, loud sigh and then smile.

Yeahhh. Great job, sister. Doesn't that feel nice? Sure does—every damn time.

2. SENSORY MEDITATION

Sensuality is all about your senses of smell, hearing, taste, sight, and touch. When we engage our senses, we heighten our awareness of pleasure.

> *"Every sexual episode starts in your senses. Whether it's a touch, a taste, a scent, a sound, or a sight, arousal begins in the brain."*
>
> ~ Barbara Carrellas[4]

Below are some ideas to tap into any/all of your senses during your meditation.

Smell: Turn on a diffuser with a few drops of ylang ylang (an aphrodisiac).

Hearing: Play groovy music or listen to water (live or on an app).

Taste: Eat or suck on something yummy before, during, or after your meditation.

Sight: Close your eyes or look at something lovely (i.e., set up a hand mirror, lie back, and gaze at your vulva).

Touch: Apply lotion to your body, massage*, masturbate, and/or rest your hands flat and wide on your low belly with fingers pointing down.

You can lie down, sit comfortably, or move gently. Once you're ready to begin, set a timer for three minutes, breathe, feel, and connect with your senses.

*Mayan abdominal massage is highly beneficial in balancing your sexual energy, as it stimulates blood flow and movement within the lower torso. I've been practicing it for about five years now. It's a whole process, but I do about a three-minute shortened version. Lying on my bed, I apply a teeny bit of coconut oil on my hands and gently rub my belly in a clockwise direction, starting at my navel and moving slowly outward toward the rib cage and pelvic bones. If I feel tenderness at any time, I pause to relax and breathe.

Pro Tip: Got something that vibrates? Use that instead of your hands.

3. INHALE, EXHALE, REPEAT

This breath technique will quite literally rock your world. No, really. I mean it. One of the members in my yoga program says she can bring herself to orgasm just by practicing this breath. How about that for a testimonial? Woot! Okay, where was I?

I call it the 3D Breath because I want your entire torso to move three-dimensionally as you breathe. (Go low. Think *vulva*.) This breath will condition the muscles and tissues of your pelvic floor so they will be more apt to respond appropriately during bedroom and bathroom habits.

- Lie supine on the floor or your bed.
- Bend your knees to bring your feet flat and (at least) hip-width apart.
- Relax your jaw, close your eyes and lips, breathe through your nose, and stay in the moment.
- On your inhale, relax and expand your belly, sides, back, and pelvic floor.
- On your exhale, engage and contract your belly, sides, back, and pelvic floor.
- Repeat for three minutes.

Have patience with yourself as you practice. This may come easily, but it may not. For maximum success, join my membership. This breath technique is the foundation for all of our practices.

4. GO WITH THE FLOW

Connect with your water element. You *are* flow.

Sing, write, dance, color, play, laugh, and yogaahhh. Below are some groovy yoga flows that tap into your emotional energy. As you practice, close your eyes and feel all the feels.

Sufi Circles: In a seated position, close your eyes and circle your torso in one direction for a minute, then switch directions and circle for another minute. Your brain state in this moving meditation is the same as when you're nearing orgasm.

Cat/Cow: On the floor (or your bed) on hands and knees, exhale as you round your back like a Halloween cat, then inhale as you lift your hips, heart, and head; repeat the flow for one minute.

Bridge Flow: In a supine position with knees bent and feet flat on the floor, practice the 3D Breath (exhale as you lift your pelvis a few inches and inhale as you lower back down). This helps to increase blood flow to the muscles surrounding the sexual organs, which helps in orgasm. Repeat this flow for one minute.

5. SPEAK YOUR TRUTH

Sex, pleasure, libido, masturbation, hormones, and leakage—some of our mothers and grandmothers never even spoke these words aloud in their entire lifetime.

To this day, taboo topics are still commonly avoided. Why are these conversations so hush-hush?

Imagine you're at Target making small talk with an acquaintance, and she mentions how badly she's struggling with vaginal dryness. What's your reaction?

Oh no, she didn't! OMG. Did anyone else hear that? What do I even say?

Even if you also struggle with vaginal dryness, chances are great this isn't a chat you're inspired to have, especially not at Target.

Somehow, these conversations trigger feelings of shame. It's like all of a sudden, we're ripped open and raw for all to see the things we don't even want to see ourselves. We judge ourselves for not knowing what to say, and we judge her for bringing up the subject in the first place! But the more we tackle taboo topics, the faster we free ourselves from the grip of them.

Don't get me wrong, I'm not suggesting you go to Target to tackle taboo topics, but I do suggest you dive into this discussion with your partner, a friend, your doctor, or me.

Simply take a deep breath, know that you're safe, then speak your truth.

One Last Thing

As I wrap up this chapter in a Florida airport after a kickass book signing this afternoon, I want to share a secret before boarding the plane home to Maryland.

These creative ways to *get your sexy back* are 100% available to you, sister. It's a practice. As you can see, it's easier than you think.

Here's the deal. I encourage you to stop saying your sex drive is **gone** or your sexuality is a thing of the past. Your sexuality will never go away, ***ever***. This is what makes you, you. This is your energy that creates life. This is your sacred feminine power! Like the rest of us, you were born with it.

Now that you know the truth, get out there and share the good news.

No, really, what are you waiting for? Get out there and share!

For more poses, breath work, and techniques specific to sexuality, chakra balancing, and fascia release, join my membership here: https://www.stretchyourspirit.com/yogainreallife

REFERENCES

1 https://www.webmd.com/sex-relationships/features/loss-of-sexual-desire-in-women

2 https://iriskrasnow.com/_pages/book_sex_after.htm

3 https://www.wsj.com/articles/the-positive-power-of-a-good-sigh-27e8f0c6

4 https://www.womenshealthnetwork.com/sexual-health/good-sex-starts-in-your-senses/

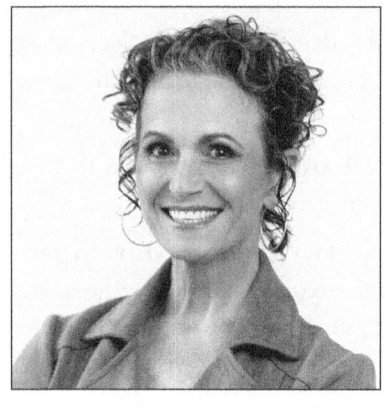

Julie Blamphin uses her positive vibe and racy authenticity to provide a personalized and intimate experience that centers around joy, stability, and sensuality.

She's an author, speaker, the founder of Stretch Your Spirit, and has been featured in *We Lead, Building Connection, Community, and Collaboration for Women in Business*; AARP The Ethel; Livestrong Magazine; The Leading Lady Podcast; Baltimore Banner; The Dr. Kinney Show; Pelvic Health Support Canada; and a long list of top podcasts and YouTube channels.

Julie can whistle like a champ, is obsessed with cartwheels and alone time, and loves to dream in Spanish.

Follow her on social media:

www.Facebook.com/StretchYourSpirit

www.Instagram.com/StretchYourSpirit

www.Linkedin.com/in/JulieBlamphin

To book Julie to speak and learn more about her and her work:

www.StretchYourSpirit.com

CHAPTER 8

Marriage, Baby, and Business, Oh my!

NAVIGATING A GOOD OPPORTUNITY WITH SEEMINGLY BAD TIMING

AliceAnne Loftus, Entrepreneur, Business and Leadership Coach

"We should do this!" I sat straight up in bed and said aloud with a certainty that startled me even though they were words coming out of my own mouth. Waking my husband, he jumps up while still tangled in bedsheets and rapid-fires anxious statements and questions, "I'll get dressed. The hospital bag is already in the car. What do you need? Are you okay?" He's clearly panicked and yet somehow prepared to get me to the labor and delivery ward in record time.

"No, no, no! I'm not in labor. I'm talking about opening a preschool! I think we should do it. I want to do it. I know we can do it. I want to start my own business."

I was speaking in short, choppy sentences, almost in disbelief at the words coming out of my mouth. This is what I was laying there thinking about at 2 a.m. just days before my due date as we're expecting our first child. Maybe I should have been thinking about the final touches on the nursery or what layette set I'd dress her in to bring her home from the hospital.

The timing was ridiculous. ludicrous, really. Insane, to say the least. Yet, there I was, not counting Braxton Hicks, but counting how many weeks I had before the official start of the school year and wondering if I could realistically be set up, ready to open my doors and welcome children to the classrooms.

He looked at me dumbfounded, possibly a little relieved, and then, with a face I had come to understand meant he was taking me very seriously, he asked, "Are you sure? We're days away from having a baby. We will have a lot of work to do. You really think you're up for this?"

I smiled, held my belly, and laid back down. I exhaled with a whisper, "This is perfect for us. I just know it."

"I'll call them first thing in the morning, and we'll get the process started," he said as he laid back down on his side, draping his hand over my hip and snuggling just a little closer to me. "Hey. Next time you feel the need to shout in the middle of the night, maybe start by telling me you're not in labor."

The truth is, I never imagined I'd be a business owner. So, how did we get to this point?

My husband and I had a whirlwind romance. From the moment we met, we knew we were in it for the long haul. I was living in Kansas City, Missouri, working in a public school for a Kindergarten enrichment program. This was back when kindergarten was still only a half day. He lived in Annapolis, Maryland, and owned his own masonry company. We met online, and within weeks, I was moving to Maryland. We had a short engagement and a beautiful wedding and were expecting a baby soon after. We had a lot happen in a very short time, and I often compare it to building a plane while learning to fly. It was a crazy time with a lot of adjustments and so many new adventures. In less than two years, I went from living in one state with a stable career to moving to a new state, getting married, and now expecting a baby. It was a lot, to say the least.

We built our life together at high speed, and while things seemed to fall into place for us, I felt a little lost; I didn't know what I wanted to do about teaching. My entire life, I had wanted to be a teacher. I loved working with kids. I was in school for elementary education, specifically special education and literacy, but when I moved to Maryland, college credits and teaching certifications didn't transfer. I had difficulty navigating where I wanted to work and how much schooling I needed to redo or complete to be able to teach in Maryland. Seriously, why is it so hard for teachers to transfer to a new state and teach? You'd think it would be easier, especially considering there's been a teacher shortage for as long as I can remember. I felt like something was missing - like I had lost a bit of my identity.

At six months pregnant, I ended up taking a job at a child care center near our home, thinking it was something I could do until our baby arrived, and then I'd have a place for her to attend so I could go back to school and get my teaching certification. I worked part-time, taking classes at the local college and prepping for her arrival all at the same time. The bigger my belly grew, so did my curiosity and perspective. I started to question what I wanted my life to look like after she arrived. I felt worn down by my part-time job because, having worked in Kindergarten enrichment before, I felt frustrated that they weren't setting up an environment that used best practices to get the children ready for Kindergarten. We were missing so many opportunities to support learning, socialization, and emotional development. My maternal instincts came in with a fierce conviction as I looked at the toddlers at my place of work and thought about what their parents would want for them. I wanted to do better. I felt that everything I was learning about early education and wanted as a new mother wasn't supported or demonstrated where I worked.

I tried many times to speak with my boss, the owner of the program, and at first she was very enthusiastic for me to implement my ideas. She even asked me to be the Director of her program. *We can make these changes! These children and families deserve better.*

However, I quickly learned that some of the changes and updates were not well received and required time, energy, and probably even money. The owner wanted to cut corners, and there were a few things she was willing to sacrifice to make more of a profit. Trust me, I don't judge her for that. It was her business. It wasn't my place to tell her how to run her business. However, something gnawed away at me. Something was telling me it wasn't right for me.

I even went to one of my professors and explained how I felt at the end of the semester. I told her that I just believed in my core that we could do more and provide better for the children and families. I learned so much from her in her class, and it affirmed everything I felt and all I believed about early childhood education.

"I just don't know what to do," I shared. "I feel so frustrated because I have seen firsthand the support children need for Kindergarten readiness and the long-term challenges they can experience without early intervention and resources. I don't think that's something I can sit back and just watch without trying my best to do better." My heart was heavy, and I started to question whether or not I could really make a difference at my job.

"Well, AliceAnne, you have two options: You can try and get her to understand the need for quality child care and implement the changes, or you can quit." She looked at me sympathetically and continued, "If you really believe in something, don't let anyone stop you. If you're seeing a need for something better, I guarantee you other parents are needing it too."

Feeling defeated and trying to focus on what was truly my responsibility (oh yeah, baby on the way!) I decided that rather than twist myself in knots over a program I was not likely going to change, I'd focus on my family. I wouldn't put my new baby in child care and I wouldn't try to get another job teaching. I'd stay home with her and apply everything I knew about early education and what I wanted as a mother and do my best for her, my family, and us.

I talked it over with my husband, and he was very supportive. While making the decision to stay home, I knew I'd want a plan to contribute something financially as well as have my own means for spending money, so I did what many do, and I signed up for a side hustle (Mary Kay) and told myself I'd build a schedule that fit around my new life as a mother. I went to work the next day and turned in my resignation.

If my story stopped there, that would be perfectly reasonable and respectable, and I hope no one would cast judgment on me or the choice we made for us at that time. I was happy with that decision. I was excited and optimistic. Aside from wanting to be a teacher, I knew I wanted to be a mother my entire life. Just ask my own mother how many baby dolls I carried around and my husband how clear I made it that I wanted to start a family immediately. Motherhood was woven into the very fiber of my being. Yet, there was a teeny tiny voice in the back of my mind that said, "Not working isn't forever, you'll find something," as I began the final weeks of my pregnancy.

Less than two weeks after I turned in my resignation, the owner of the program announced she was closing the business. As families came to pick up their children from child care on a Friday afternoon, she informed them they wouldn't have child care the following Monday. You read that right; less than seventy-two hours of notice were given to families to find alternative child care. It was a disaster. Complete chaos ensued. Families were left scrambling, frustrated, feeling abandoned, and shocked that they now were left looking at a frantic weekend ahead, calling family, friends, and anyone who could possibly help and still not likely to find long-term options for child care to be able to return to work on Monday.

All the employees had just learned they were also out of a job. To say that everyone was left feeling blindsided would be the understatement of the year. I stood there like a deer in headlights, watching everything fall apart and wondering how things could've turned south so quickly. I was also relieved that I hadn't placed my bets that I'd have a job to return to after our baby was born. I felt horrible for the staff, families, and children, but immense relief that it wasn't my problem. I know that sounds callous, but honestly, I felt like I dodged a bullet, and I found comfort in knowing I wasn't going to be part of the aftermath of this disaster as I'd blissfully start the next chapter of my life without having to clean up this mess.

Or so I thought.

When I got home that afternoon, my phone was ringing off the hook. Employees and parents were calling me to vent, cry, ask for help, and cry some more. Even though my time as Director of the program was very short, since the owner was not accepting phone calls nor was she willing to have any discussions with anyone regarding the matter, my guess is that I was the next person they thought to call.

"I cannot believe this is happening! What is our family going to do?" a parent cried.

"How am I going to find a new job now? Will I even be able to get a reference since she closed the business? Is that something you can help me with?" a former coworker pleaded. "What are we all going to do?"

I'm going to have a baby, I thought. *This isn't really my issue.*

I was listening to them and realizing that a simple Band-Aid solution would be to connect them together and see if they could help each other out. Even though it wasn't really my problem to solve, the solution was so clear and made so much sense I figured it wouldn't hurt to try and help. I started calling all the staff and asking them if they would be willing to connect with the families and create some sort of temporary care where they could watch groups of children in the families' homes. Obviously, we weren't able to help everyone, but we had enough staff and families willing to pull together to help the most desperate families get immediate temporary care and help the newly unemployed still receive income while they were trying to find a new job.

Good thinking, AliceAnne. I felt happy with how I was able to help. I could walk away knowing I did all I could—until the phone rang again.

"Hi, AliceAnne Loftus? This is Fred. I'm the owner of the building of Safe Harbor Child Care. I heard you were helping everyone, and I have a proposition."

What was he saying? Am I hearing this right? Is he asking me to buy the building?

"Hello? Mrs. Loftus? I'm not interested in being a landlord anymore. I'd be willing to give you an incredible deal on the building as long as you promise to open a childcare center. The community really needs this. It's been a childcare program for the last 30 years. I don't know what the community would do without it. Will you think about it?" he continued.

In complete disbelief, I respond to him, "Thank you so much for thinking of me. I don't think I'm the right person for this. I'm about to have a baby in just a few weeks or days even, and I don't know the first thing about running a business. I'm a teacher. Let me just wrap my head around this and see if I know of anyone who would be willing to take you up on this offer." I hung up and couldn't stop thinking about his words for several days. *Was this something I could do?*

That night, when I woke my husband up declaring my decision that I was, in fact, going to buy a building and start a business, the course of our lives changed drastically. Would I recommend that someone move states, get married, get pregnant, and start a business within such a short time frame? Probably not. Do we really have control of the timing of things? Certainly not. At least we do not control the timing of when opportunities present themselves. There were so many moments with my husband that I thought, *this is terrible timing*. Yet, jumping feet first seemed to be exactly what I needed to do to take that next brave step.

The next several days were an absolute blur. We bought the property and had so many meetings: the Department of Education, lawyers, and doctors; we had a baby at 8:41 a.m. one morning, and my husband had to quickly scoot out to meet a contractor for our renovations at 10 a.m. I swaddled and nursed while conducting interviews and picking out new furniture (not for my own baby, but for the new toddler classrooms). My father-in-law sanded and sealed the playground equipment while my mother-in-law held our baby girl so I could finalize our website. I think back on those early days with tears in my eyes, as both my in-laws have now passed, and I hope they know just how grateful I am for their support.

My mother cooked in my kitchen and bathed our baby so I could sleep, shower, and prepare myself for our licensing inspection. My husband worked round the clock with contractors and spent every waking moment getting the building ready for our opening day. My milk let down in an important meeting with my licensing specialist, and I think she took pity on me and cut the meeting short while granting my variance request to bring my newborn baby with me to my new preschool center, even though my license was for children ages two through five.

Eight weeks after that night, I declared my decision and opened the doors to my new preschool center. I had eight teachers employed (many from the previous center that closed), six children enrolled, and one newborn baby in a Bjorn on my chest. We're coming up on our twentieth anniversary in business. I raised both my children there. I even opened a second location when my second child was a toddler. I have had the most fulfilling career and didn't miss a minute with my own children. I built a business with the brain of an educator and the heart of a mother. I took my skills, knowledge, and passion and created something that fit my family. I relied on my resources and support systems and figured out how to make things work. I didn't give up on my convictions, and as I look back on the last twenty years and think that it was the worst timing ever, and it was absolutely perfect, I know that sometimes you can't plan or schedule when things will work out, you just have to trust yourself and never give up on what you believe.

THE TOOL

Do you find yourself at a crossroads of good opportunity and tough timing? Here are some journal prompts to help you navigate the decision process.

1. WHAT DO YOU WANT YOUR LIFE TO LOOK LIKE?

....
....
....
....

2. WHAT ARE YOUR CORE VALUES? WHAT IS IMPORTANT TO YOU PERSONALLY? WHAT IS IMPORTANT TO YOU FOR YOUR FAMILY?

....
....
....
....

3. WHAT SKILLS AND TALENTS DO YOU POSSESS?

....
....
....
....

4. WHAT ARE YOUR RESOURCES AND SUPPORT SYSTEMS?

....
....
....
....

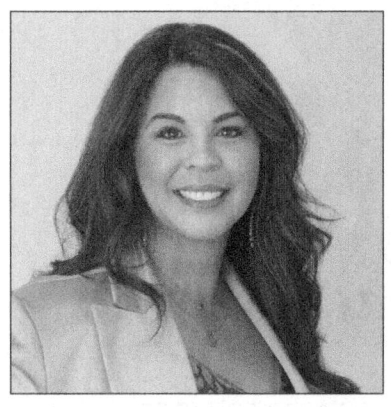

AliceAnne Loftus is the founder of Bright Beginning Children's Learning Center (2004) as well as Leading Lady Coaching (2016). With two decades of experience as an entrepreneur, community leader, public speaker, and author, she has devoted her life to helping women feel empowered, inspired, and in the lead of their own lives. She resides in Annapolis, Maryland with her husband. Their daughter, now in college, and son, in high school, have been at the center of their businesses, and it is with great pride that they have also developed incredible work ethics and intrinsic drives to create their own paths. When AliceAnne isn't thinking up new business strategies and ideas, you'll find her building puzzles, traveling, cooking up a storm, or binge-watching terrible TV.

Learn more about AliceAnne at www.leadinglady-coaching.com and www.bright-beginning.com

Join https://www.facebook.com/groups/LeadingLadiesAAL to connect with other high-achieving women in business and leadership

Follow https://www.instagram.com/leading.lady.coach and https://www.instagram.com/bbclc/

Read We Lead https://a.co/d/cdtvhtA and Take the Lead https://a.co/d/8Il0a4r

CHAPTER 9

Your Body Has Changed

HONOR IT WITH CURIOSITY AND REST

Dr. Gina Hahn, DPT, RKC

MY STORY

I was relieved and disappointed at the same time. I was grateful my baby was healthy, and grieving the birth I wanted.

I woke up in the recovery room, groggy and concerned.

"Is he okay?" I asked.

"Yes, he's perfect," my husband replied with a smile. He was holding our newborn son skin to skin.

Thank God.

I had so many questions. *Why was his heart rate low during labor? What else could we have tried? Was my body the problem? Why did this happen to me? Was the c-section absolutely necessary? Would I be able to have a vaginal birth in the future?*

I was spiraling.

I wanted, planned, and prepared for an unmedicated home birth. I wanted to be in my nest and bring my baby into a calm, warm, familiar environment. I trusted my body. I learned as much as I could about labor through the Bradlee Method birthing classes, podcasts like Evidence Based Birth, and conversations with other women who had unmedicated births. My husband did, too. We were a united front and we were making informed decisions together. It was a beautiful time in our life.

I felt empowered during my pregnancy. I wanted to be a pioneer among my group of friends. A small part of me wanted to prove something to them and to myself.

"Can I hold him?" I asked.

"Not yet," the anesthesiologist said.

I felt out of control. I was also high from the anesthesia.

I just want to hold him. I would feel better if I held him.

I bawled on the car ride home two days later. I was devastated. I had failed.

My body failed.

Touching my wound, which was stapled shut, was incredibly challenging and emotional. It felt like it didn't belong to me. The whole experience didn't belong to me for a long time. I couldn't relate to what had unfolded.

It was ten days before they took the staples out, it took another year to heal the invisible wounds. The disappointment and grief were pervasive. I tried to affirm myself and my body over and over again. I tried to get to a place of acceptance and maybe even gratitude. I also went to therapy.

Thank you (my body) for growing, carrying, and birthing this baby.

Thank you for my healthy boy.

I am badass for having this scar.

Physically, my body healed well and without complications. I was grateful for that. I attribute this to prioritizing rest for two weeks immediately postpartum (more to come on that later), as well as my commitment to weight training, weekly walks, hydration, and a diet rich in protein throughout my pregnancy.

This was the experience that launched me into pelvic floor physical therapy (PT).

I was first introduced to pelvic floor PT in graduate school when I injured my tailbone. My professor referred me to a physical therapist who specializes in pelvic floor health. She manipulated my tailbone intravaginally, and I could sit again without pain. It was a significant change in my day-to-day life.

After graduation, I took a traditional route into physical therapy practice. I worked with folks recovering from injuries and surgeries and quickly learned that movement and (heavy) load were the most impactful for rehabilitation.

People feel fragile, weak, and scared in the presence of pain and injury, and my role was to help them feel strong and capable again in a safe environment. All of this is also true during pregnancy and the postpartum period, which for many is about 6 to 12 months long.

Here I was, a new mom with a background in PT, traumatized and determined to give my birth story a new meaning. I decided to leverage my expertise to help women understand and trust their bodies, assure them it is not a failure if things don't go as planned, and provide a path forward to feeling resilient.

Fast forward to my second pregnancy. Our son was over two years old. I spent nine months working on my emotional readiness for this labor. I journaled, meditated, hired a doula, exercised, talked about my fears and doubts, and scheduled routine counseling sessions.

My body is strong.

My body knows how to birth this baby.

My baby knows how to be born to me.

Breathe deep.

Go inward.

These affirmations were not only internal. I wrote them down in my prettiest handwriting and pasted them around my home office.

My preference was to have an unmedicated delivery and a VBAC (vaginal birth after cesarean). I spoke with my providers about my trauma associated with being put under anesthesia for my first birth (which was necessary for a quick delivery, as I arrived at the hospital fully dilated, pushing, and my baby had low fetal heart tones).

My providers assured me, "Because you will labor and deliver in the hospital, there will be *time* to get an epidural or spinal if a repeat c-section is necessary."

I wanted to be awake to greet my baby this time.

One Friday afternoon in December, my water broke. I was so excited! I was ready. Whatever was about to happen, I would ride the wave.

The next morning, nineteen hours later, I pushed my daughter through my body and into this world with everything I had. It was powerful.

I did it!

My body did it.

My baby, she's here.

That was the most primal thing I've ever done. I felt everything in those fleeting moments. Sure, there was pain, but I expected that. I felt triumphant.

Again, I required stitches, but this time for a first-degree tear of my labia, which was minor in comparison to the cesarean. I wanted to look at and touch this wound, different from my c-section experience. This time, I was curious and proud.

During pregnancy, a person changes physically and emotionally, most of which happens without conscious effort, which is pretty cool. Generally, our bodies progress through pregnancy and labor without issues, but it's important to get regular checkups and to be informed and prepared for risks associated with pregnancy and delivery.

In postpartum recovery, our bodies still know what to do, whether it's healing from a cesarean or a vaginal birth. The best thing you can do in those first few weeks is set up the right environment for healing: rest, hydration, and nourishment (also important throughout pregnancy).

I know not all cesarean births are traumatic and that not all vaginal births are triumphant. This is my story. Your story will be different and unique to you.

I want *you* to know that your body was designed to open and has the wisdom to knit itself back together again.

You're not alone. If you work at it, you will heal and find your strength again.

THE TOOL

INITIAL STEPS TO SUPPORT YOUR HEALING

The first step is how to set the stage for optimal healing. The second step is to be curious about the changes.

Step 1: Rest. The most productive thing you can do in the first two weeks postpartum is *rest*. Set this as your expectation, and communicate it to your partner.

This means:

- No walks in the first two weeks. Just because you *can* doesn't mean you should.
- Limit stair climbing to two times per day. Come down in the morning; go up in the evening.
- Rest with your hips up for 20 minutes two times a day. Lie down on your back with your knees bent, lift your butt, and prop your hips on a pillow or folded blanket. This helps with swelling management.
- Use compression garments like postpartum leggings and a belly binder.

These rules apply whether you had a cesarean or a vaginal delivery.

If your baby is not home with you, you're probably making trips to and from the hospital. Compression garments will be important for you. Ask to be dropped off at the front door instead of walking from the parking garage. If there is a wheelchair, use it.

Pay attention to your need for rest, hydration, and nourishment. These are foundational to restoration but can be easily ignored. Give yourself grace.

Give yourself a license to just be. Your daily productivity is going to look different. Your new to-do list should read "Do less."

Step 2: Before your six-week check-up, look at yourself in a full-length mirror and with a hand mirror. Don't be in a rush.

Let's start with your lower abdomen. Lift and move tissue up as needed to support visualization.

In the first six weeks postpartum, if you have a c-section scar, it should be dry and pink in color. It probably has an irregular texture, not smooth. It's likely taut and puckering instead of flat or uniform. The skin and scar might be warm to the touch. This area is likely tender. Get a feel for it now, and check again over the next few days and weeks to feel progress.

Okay, now grab a hand mirror, and allow me to walk you through a self-exam of your vulva and vagina. You can choose to stand with one leg up, or you can sit reclined with both knees bent.

I'm scared. I have never looked with a hand mirror before.

You're so brave! Your whole body is amazing.

Let's identify the following structures:

- Labia majora
- Labia minora
- Clitoris and clitoral hood
- Urethral opening
- Vaginal opening and vaginal canal
- Anus

Okay, deep breath, we're going for it.

Angle the mirror so you can see your vulva. You have two outer lips called labia majora. This is where your pubic hair typically grows. There are two inner lips called labia minora, which might actually extend beyond labia majora, and that is perfectly normal. The labia minora do not have hair and are often asymmetrical.

Spread your labia majora to view the clitoris and clitoral hood (the skin that surrounds the clitoris). This is your pleasure zone. In fact, embryologically, this tissue is the same as the head or glans of the penis. It's packed with lots of nerve endings for pleasure. Only a small part is external; there are internal 'legs' of the clitoris that we cannot see that extend all the way to the vaginal opening. The whole clitoris (what we can and cannot see) becomes engorged or swells with blood during arousal, similar to how a penis becomes erect.

With your labia still spread, observe your vaginal opening. Lift up slightly to reveal your urethral opening, from which you urinate. It's typically tucked away in the moist microbiome of your vagina, which keeps it free from bacteria and infection.

The vagina or vaginal canal is incredibly adaptable. It typically sits closed like a sock that just came out of the dryer. When something is inserted, the vagina opens or envelopes the shape and size of said object. It's amazing! It's designed to stretch and heal very well.

Lastly, observe your anus. If you try a pelvic floor contraction or kegel, you should see your anus wink and your clitoris nod. That just means movement. This is something I would look for during a pelvic exam.

Well, what do you think?

If you're like me, you think it's all pretty cool. The human body is fascinating!

You might notice some changes, like sutures, if you had a tear or extra folds of tissue. Don't be alarmed. What you see is likely normal adaptations to a) carrying a baby for nine months and b) birthing a baby.

Even if you had a cesarean, there might be changes in your vagina because you did, in fact, grow a baby in your body, so tissue and organs shifted to allow that to happen. Also, many moms have a trial of labor before needing or deciding to have a cesarean (like I did), so things stretch.

You should see a specialist if you have symptoms that are interfering with your physical or mental well-being, such as:

- The incision site is red, swollen, or opened
- Yellow or green drainage from either your c-section site or your vulva if you had a tear
- Splotchy skin or rash-like skin changes
- Urine leakage (incontinence)
- Changes in bowel movements (feeling incomplete emptying, leaking bowels, pressure, etc)
- Feelings of pressure or heaviness in your vulva/vagina
- Pain with sex, specifically intercourse
- And others

Scar tissue should be addressed by a specialist even if you don't have symptoms. It is important to massage and stretch the tissue surrounding the scar as well as the scar itself so that it moves freely with the rest of your skin and the structures underneath.

If you have symptoms interfering with your self-confidence or quality of life, don't guess; get assessed.

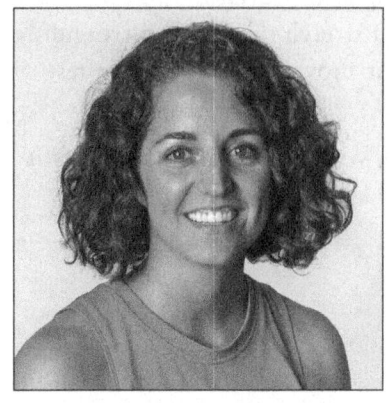

Dr. Gina Hahn, DPT, RKC, is an expert pelvic floor physical therapist. She helps people reconnect with their pleasure and joy, even in the presence of pain and injury. She spent the early part of her career in strength and conditioning, helping clients feel resilient in their bodies and get back into the gym. She chose the pelvic floor as a specialty following her first pregnancy. She realized the need for and value of this specialization as she moved through an adverse event and came out stronger on the other side. Gina empowers clients and helps them feel fully seen and heard, moving seamlessly from health care provider to coach, to integrate and address the mind-body-soul of each client for effective and long-lasting results. Expect to lift weights, breathe, move, and do things that don't seem possible. She helps her clients to see *they* are the experts of their bodies, and she will coach you on how to tune in and connect with your own powerful inner healer. When Gina is off duty, you'll find her reflecting on the joys and challenges of loving two children and supporting their growth and development with her husband, dancing in the front row at a concert, or reading in her hammock under the trees.

Connect with Dr. Gina:

Website: https://www.ginaperformancetherapy.com/

Instagram: https://www.instagram.com/performxtherapy/

CHAPTER 10

Motherhood Is Hard. Eating Doesn't Have to Be.

HEALTHY EATING SIMPLIFIED

Elizabeth Harris, MS, RDN, Certified Intuitive Eating Counselor

MY STORY

The summer before my senior year of high school, my world changed quite substantially almost overnight. It started with a hitch in the spot just below my middle finger in the palm of one of my hands. My finger felt like it was catching at that spot and I couldn't fully straighten it. *Weird and annoying, but whatever.* I continued hanging at the beach with my then-boyfriend.

Days later, though, I noticed that all my fingers were swollen. Within a week or so, I had puffy lumps popping up elsewhere in my body. There may have been pain or aching, but to be honest, the thing I remember the most is the swelling and the limited mobility it caused.

"Mom, something's wrong."

And so began a battery of doctor appointments, blood tests, and sick days from school. It didn't take long before I was diagnosed with rheumatoid arthritis (RA). At my lowest point, I had swelling, some the size of golf balls or bigger, in nearly every joint in my body—even my jaw.

Arthritis, I thought, *isn't that for old people? And what happens now? I'm in pain, and everything is so swollen that I can't move right.*

In case you're not familiar, rheumatoid arthritis is an inflammatory autoimmune condition that affects the lining of your joints and can eventually cause bone deterioration or joint deformity. It's not limited to just your joints, though; it can also impact your eyes, heart, and lungs, among other tissues. So yeah, it's not an age-related disease, and it's scary to get that diagnosis at such a young age.

We were fortunate enough to live within about an hour's drive from Yale New Haven Hospital in Connecticut, where they had renowned doctors specializing in rheumatology and RA. Here's what I remember most from the next 12 months: long drives back and forth into the city, usually weekly; having blood drawn more times than I ever thought possible; getting weekly shots of gold (yes, actual shots of gold, which was one of the RA treatments at the time); trying a slew of other medications, some of which resulted in allergic reactions that caused me to break out in full-body hives; and eventually, taking heavy-duty steroids.

I hated the never-ending blood draws, but the steroids were the worst.

If you've ever taken prolonged, high levels of prednisone, you know it comes with a range of potential negative, annoying, and even scary side effects. Things like mood changes, vision problems, difficulty thinking, increased appetite, and dizziness, with the long-term possibility of damaging liver or kidney function.

The two side effects most difficult to deal with as a vulnerable teenager preparing for prom, graduation, and college were facial hair growth and something they call a moon face, which is exactly as it sounds. Your face gets very round, puffy, and moon-shaped. There's nothing inherently wrong with having a round, full face, of course, but when that's not your natural state (my face is long and narrow), it can really complicate your self-image and confidence, especially at such a vulnerable time in life.

Why can't I just be normal and do normal teenage things? I remember wishing.

LUCKY, WITH A SIDE OF MOTHERHOOD

As much as I hated all the invasive treatments, they worked. By the time I was heading off to college, my RA was mostly in remission and well-managed with low-level medications. My fingers would occasionally swell and get stiff, but that was the primary symptom I dealt with. I remember the doctor saying that, in the best-case scenario, it could turn out to be juvenile RA that may never return. Time would tell.

Unfortunately for me, that wasn't the case. My RA has plagued me on and off throughout my life, and yet, I still consider myself to be very, very lucky. Here's why.

Sometime during college, I weaned myself off even those low-level meds, and my RA was mostly in the background of my life until I became a mom in my late twenties. However, after each one of my three babies was born, I had a significant flare-up.

The first one sent me back to a rheumatologist for the first time in ten years or so. I lived in a different state and was seeing a different doctor, but after reviewing all my history, he wanted to put me back on prednisone.

No, no, no; I really, really don't want to have to do that. Not now. Not again. I'm breastfeeding.

"Thank you," I said, "I'll think about it and see how my joints feel over the next few weeks."

Inside, I felt desperate to find any other solution. I decided to see an acupuncturist to see if it might help. "I think I can help you, but it's going to take multiple treatments and lots of patience," he told me. I got a babysitter for my infant daughter and began going to acupuncture two times per week for about six months. In addition to the treatments, he advised me to change some things in my diet and prescribed some awful-tasting Chinese herbs.

I did everything he recommended, paying careful attention to my diet and lifestyle choices. I was fully committed to seeing if an alternative treatment path could work.

Eventually, my flareup fully subsided without medications or steroids. I had similar flareups after each of my next two babies were born, and I continued with healthy eating and acupuncture, although fewer and fewer treatments were necessary to get it under control each time.

I now know that hormonal shifts play a big role in my RA; case in point, I'm dealing with another significant bout of active RA now that I'm solidly in perimenopause.

Over the years, whenever I've had a minor flare-up, I head back to my acupuncturist. I buckle down, adhering even more closely than usual to my anti-inflammatory eating pattern. I've never been a big drinker, but I stop having wine altogether as I know it exacerbates my inflammation. I pour more energy into the ways I'm taking care of myself and my body.

I've been extremely lucky that my RA responds to these practices very well. However, I want to be clear and upfront that I'm fully aware not everyone with RA, other autoimmune conditions, or diseases will see such positive results without (or, frankly, even with) serious medications or other more invasive treatments. *Maybe I should have titled this section Lucky, With a Heaping Side of Gratitude?*

ANOTHER MAJOR LIFE TRANSITION

I didn't go off to college and study anything related to health. To be honest, I was a bit shellshocked by my diagnosis and the difficult treatment year that followed; also, as one of the first people in my family to go to college, I had absolutely no idea or direction for what I wanted to do with my life. Plus, it would take a lot more time for me to understand I could have an active role in managing my disease instead of just feeling like a helpless victim.

Still, my experience with RA at such a pivotal time in my development has had a profound impact on my career, belief system, and the direction my life would eventually take. I learned from a relatively early age just how important and fragile health is. I didn't do anything to cause my RA, but I lived through the impact (including the pain, medications, side effects, life disruptions, and fear) of losing my health.

I learned not to take health for granted but to view it as a precious gift to be safeguarded to whatever extent possible.

As Herophilus, an early Greek physician, is said to have stated, "When health is absent, wisdom cannot reveal itself, art cannot become manifest, strength cannot be exerted, wealth is useless, and reason is powerless."

RA taught me to be proactive about looking after my body. It taught me the importance of nutrition, exercise, rest, stress management, preventative medical care, and being your own dogged advocate for and champion promoter of your health.

It also sparked an interest in and passion for nutrition, exercise, and overall wellness. Eventually, after contemplating it for many, many years and doing a long stint as a stay-at-home mom, I made a complete career switch and went back to school in my 40s to get a Master's degree in nutrition science and become a licensed, registered dietitian nutritionist (RDN).

My goal? To work in health promotion, inspiring and teaching people to improve or promote their eating, health, and wellbeing with flexible, enjoyable nutrition and other health-promoting lifestyle choices. There's something fundamentally different about my approach to nutrition and health that I can't wait to share with you in just a minute.

BUT FIRST, A LOVE LETTER TO MOMS EVERYWHERE

It turns out it's no small endeavor to become a dietitian, especially when you have a Bachelor of Arts degree in Russian language and very little background in the sciences! I had to take thirteen pre-requisite science courses just to get into the master's program at the University of Southern California, a couple of which I'd already taken during my undergrad program twenty years earlier.

It took me so long to get through these prereq courses, mostly one by one due to their sequential nature, that the validity of one even expired before I could apply to the program, forcing me to take it a second time.

Once accepted to the program, I had to secure and complete eight different dietetic internship rotations (trust me, this is more difficult than it sounds as there's a national shortage of willing dietetic preceptors and I had no university connections or assistance since I was a distance student on the opposite coast). I did it all while completing the coursework for my degree *and raising three active adolescents.*

To say this was a difficult and stressful undertaking would be an understatement. It's honestly one of the hardest things I've ever done, motherhood aside.

I don't talk about this much but before each new dietetic rotation, we received a booklet of the required dietetic competencies and associated assignments for that rotation. Every single time I received that workbook, I mean literally for every single one of the eight internship rotations, I looked at it and thought, *there is absolutely no way I can do this. It's too hard. It will take too much time. I'm forty years old; why the hell am I interning anywhere? I shouldn't be spending this valuable time away from my kids.*

On and on, my self-doubt and negative self-talk went. Even after I'd completed seven other rotations, I thought the same thing about number eight, with my brain trying to convince me to give up and play it safe.

That's BS, I would tell myself. *Look around you, you're the oldest person by far in this program. Most of these people are in their twenties. If they can do this, so can you. Think about the life experience and wisdom you have on them. You got the rotation; that's the hard part. Keep going. You're not just doing this for you. You're also doing it for your kids, to show them it's never too late to change gears, to follow your dreams, to work hard for something you want. You have something essential you want to share with the world.*

Fortunately, I successfully talked myself off the ledge each time, completing my 1200 hours of supervised dietetics practice along with my master's coursework. Two out of my three children (one was competing in a national high school sailing regatta that weekend) saw me walk down the aisle to get my diploma. All of my children have witnessed me studying, interning, switching careers, starting a successful business, becoming a published author, and helping to transform people's health and lives for the better.

Those things mean the world to me. But I do hope there's one other enduring legacy from my experience. I hope they all will know beyond a shadow of a doubt that their dreams matter. They are worthy of going after them no matter how difficult it is or what point they're at in their lives.

No matter which twisting, winding, daunting paths motherhood takes you down, I hope you'll remember the same. Your dreams matter. You deserve to go after them. And you can do hard things.

THE FORGOTTEN PART OF HEALTHY EATING

My experience with RA taught me the importance of cherishing, advocating for, and, to the extent that we're able, safeguarding our health. My education armed me with a deep appreciation and understanding of nutrition science and the human body. Subsequently, my work as a dietitian completely transformed the way I think about and approach food and health forever.

As soon as I began working in the field of nutrition, it became painfully clear to me that there was a major problem. Toxic diet culture runs rampant.

As a culture, we seem to focus far more on the pursuit of thinness than the promotion of sound nutrition and genuine health. There's tremendous fearmongering around food. People are made to feel ashamed or morally superior based on their food choices or body shape and size. Exercise is viewed primarily as a means of burning calories or "paying" for what we eat rather than a way to enrich and enhance our lives.

Meanwhile, healthy eating has been reduced to a host of extreme or rigid dieting "rules" that often conflict with or aren't supported by nutrition science. Celebrities, influencers, and average Joes think they're qualified to give nutrition guidance simply because they eat or have lost weight (usually temporarily; the research is crystal clear that dieting doesn't produce long-term, sustainable weight loss the vast majority of the time) with their latest diet. Disordered eating is not just commonplace; it's often unrecognized, normalized, and even praised in diet culture. Eating disorders, with the second highest mortality rate among all mental illnesses at present, are unfortunately on the rise.

We forget that healthy bodies come in all shapes and sizes and that body diversity and bodies changing throughout our lives are not just okay but normal. The result?

Far too many people are left feeling confused, stressed out, overwhelmed, or just plain stuck when it comes to food or their body image. This doesn't enhance health; it detracts from it.

My biggest lesson as a dietitian working predominantly with women who have battled food and their bodies for years or even decades is that it doesn't have to be this way.

Nutrients and eating patterns matter, of course. So, too, does our relationship with food and our bodies. How we eat is just as important as what we eat. Health is so much more complex than the calories on our plates or the number we see on the scale.

When we zoom out to look at our whole health (that sweet spot where physical, mental, and emotional wellbeing are all nurtured and promoted) and when we approach food through the lens of trying to care for our bodies rather than simply attempting to control our weight, healthy eating becomes simple, flexible, and yes, even enjoyable. No toxic diet culture needed.

THE TOOL

Here's my recipe for simplifying nutrition, especially as a new mom.

First and foremost, remember that your needs matter! A well-fed mom is a well-nourished mom with more energy and greater bandwidth for dealing with stress. Eat.

Know that your body is wise. If you're feeling hungry, that's your body sending you an important message about a critical need. Rather than trying to count calories (or points or macros), which disconnects you from your body's hunger and fullness cues, practice tuning into and honoring those innate body signals instead.

If you've recently given birth and are breastfeeding, your energy and nutrient needs are increased. You'll likely need at least five or six smaller meals or snacks per day. Reach out to your dietitian or doctor if you're curious about specific, increased nutrient needs during this critical period.

The basics of good nutrition go a long way:

There are three macronutrients: protein, carbs, and fat. Try to include at least two of the three in a meal or snack to make it well-balanced and satisfying. Bonus: this strategy works great for feeding toddlers and kids, too; plus, it can relieve the pressure from feeling like you must cook an elaborate meal for it to "count" as good nutrition.

Make your plates as colorful as you can by adding a variety of fruits and vegetables.

Speaking of adding, this is a great way to approach nutrition overall. Instead of stressing over which foods you *shouldn't* eat, consider what you'd like to eat and what sounds good, and then ask yourself, "How can I add nutrient-dense foods to this meal?"

Drink water and remember that other liquids count toward your hydration needs, too, including the water from fruits and veggies, tea, coffee, soups, and other beverages.

Don't let perfect be the enemy of the good. Shortcuts, such as prewashed and chopped fruits and veggies, canned beans, frozen rice, frozen fruits and veggies, pre-cooked grains, rotisserie chicken and other pre-cooked proteins, bagged salads, and other ready-made options can be very helpful.

Time is short as a new mom, so embrace flexibility and creativity. Cook when you can, even if it's early in the day. Make things you can eat at different meals in different ways or choose dishes that stretch into other meals, such as soup, pasta, rice and beans, casseroles, whole chickens, and the like.

Lastly, don't forget vitamin joy—enjoying your food is health-promoting, too!

Bonus: When your kids see you enjoying a wide variety of foods guilt-free without focusing on weight (or making critical comments about your body shape or size) you'll be sowing the seeds for them to live with food and body confidence for life!

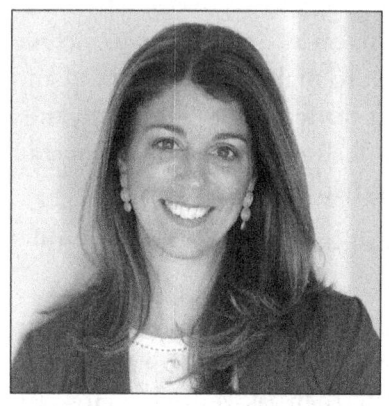

Elizabeth Harris is a registered dietitian, certified Intuitive Eating counselor, speaker, entrepreneur, and co-host of the podcast Wellness Rebranded. She's passionate about empowering people to drop out of diet culture and reimagine their relationship with food, movement, and their bodies so they can prioritize their whole health with Intuitive Eating, gentle nutrition, and body image healing.

Known for her undying love of dark chocolate peanut butter cups and compassionate, non-judgmental approach, Elizabeth's motto is "self-care, not self-control." Because food is meant to be enjoyed, movement should make you happy, and we've all got better things to do than counting carbs or calories!

Elizabeth holds a Master's degree in Nutrition, Healthspan, and Longevity from the University of Southern California and a Bachelor's degree in Russian language and Slavic and East European Studies from the University of Connecticut. In her spare time, you'll find her keeping backyard bees, gardening, reading voraciously, and traveling the world with her husband and three teenagers—hitting every available farmers' market along the way.

Follow on social media:

IG: @ElizabethHarrisNutrition

FB: @ElizabethHarrisNutrition

Join Elizabeth's Facebook Community:

www.facebook.com/groups/healthandhealingwithintuitiveeating/

Visit on the web:

www.elizabethharrisnutrition.com

Book a free whole health strategy session with Elizabeth:

https://elizabethharrisnutrition.com/booking

CHAPTER 11

Cultivating a Village

THE SUPPORT PARENTS WANT, BUT CHILDREN NEED

Tomika Robertson

Picture this. You have this amazing little human being or human beings; they're perfect in every way. But you're getting closer to returning to work.

Or life after children has been busier than expected. With soccer, tea parties, baseball, and more, keeping up with your children's schedule has taken a toll on your energy and time.

Let's face it, Mom: YOU NEED HELP!

We are all beautiful, amazing, and capable women, but a couple of pairs of extra hands would make life less hectic, right?

An old African proverb reads, "Omwana taba womoi." It translates to mean a child is not raised by one parent or house alone. This is said to be where the phrase "It takes a village to raise a child" stems from.

Think about it: when you grew up, you likely had other active people in your life who you saw regularly and assisted with your upbringing. Was it a grandmother, an auntie, an uncle, a family friend, or a neighbor? That was the village that helped raise you.

Unfortunately, our "villages" look a lot different from when our parents were raising us, but they're just as important today as they were back then.

MY STORY

At the tender age of 25, my mother found herself as a single mom with two children under the age of 3 years old. My Father died unexpectedly at a time when they had just set out on their own with a bright future ahead of them.

My Mom was forced to survive the circumstances that were handed to her. To do so she created a village that supported all of us over the years.

My great-grandmother, Mama Jill, was a main staple in the village I grew up in. We went to her house often on weekends but were dropped off at the school where she was a kindergarten teacher. Growing up, I watched her lovingly teach, love, and correct children who didn't belong to her. I saw her speak with parents, collaborate with other educators, and plan fun activities for children. In fact, I would help her prepare for fun things like breakfast with Santa, make bulletin boards, and even label shelves in her classroom. I knew at seven years old that I wanted to be an educator, just like her.

Today, as an educator and a childcare business owner, I too am a pillar in villages children are growing up in…

I get to see first-hand how stressed out and panicked most moms can be when it comes to returning to work or seeking help with all the things we, as matriarchs, are responsible for.

Almost weekly in my preschool and early learning centers, I receive calls that absolutely break my heart. An unsuspecting mom seeking childcare in our programs (because we are amazing) only to be told that we have a waiting list for a particular program or spaces won't be available until three to six months from the present day and time they're calling.

"What am I going to do?" this mom asks as the baby cries in the background and the older child, who sounds two, maybe three years old, yells, "Mommy, Mommy, Mommy," in the background. She slightly whispers, "I go back to work next month, and everyone I call has no spaces available, others not until next year."

Sobs fill the empty space as I listen and prepare to comfort this momma the best way I know how: to introduce her to other options available to her as a parent, to encourage her to join our waiting list and hold space for the words of encouragement and resources it may take to help this mom move towards the next steps of finding what her family needs—HELP!

"If you want to go fast, go alone; if you want to go far, go together."
~ African Proverb

THE TOOL
CONSTRUCTING YOUR VILLAGE

Before I dole out any resources or offer any advice, I always encourage a mom in this headspace to first breathe.

Finding trustworthy help is a marathon, not a sprint, although depending on the stage you're in, it may feel like a ten-yard dash! This usually brings a small chuckle. Now, I can move forward in helping this parent with hopefully helpful resources they need to build a village of support for their family.

Here are some of those same resources in a three-step process to cultivate a village of your own!

STEP 1: OUTLINE YOUR VILLAGE

The Pillars

The basis of your village is the details that first need attention. These details may seem small, yet they are pillars of your village.

Schedules: What are your scheduling needs? What are your written-in-stone work hours, school hours, training hours, etc.? Where do you need help meeting these scheduling needs?

I suggest writing everyone's schedule out in detail to help you see the pieces of this giant puzzle before adding additional pieces to it. Google Calendar is a great tool to use for this. You can individualize each person's schedule, color coding it for easier access and use. Another great way to accomplish this is a good old-fashioned paper planner using pencils and cute pens. The real goal is to identify all your family's unique scheduling needs and identify where the gaps are.

Before finalizing your schedule, consider discussing your schedule with your employer. Most managers know the challenges of finding childcare, and some may know from first-hand experience. Speak with your employer to see what, if anything, can be changed for even a short period while everyone is adjusting.

My motto is, if you never ask, you will never know the answer!

Next is the people.

The People

Finding people you can trust to help in times of need is crucial to your village. This would be a great time to speak with friends and family to see who can be available to help. Other moms on your child's sports teams, parents of your child's classmates, and maybe even a trusted neighbor would be willing to help during these times. Even if it's only for the one day you're running late, or your child needs an early pickup, this will be extremely important in helping build your village and put the pieces of your puzzle together.

At some point, you'll need to pull on your support system; knowing who they are and establishing these possibilities now will help you manage everything and continue to put this giant puzzle together.

In high school, my best friend's grandmother, "Mamma," was a part of my village. Momma always had snacks and candy for us whenever we came over. But she always had a word of encouragement or a stern word of fear to make sure I was staying out of trouble while my mother was working. She passed away this morning, and I write this in honor of her being a part of the village I grew up in!

STEP 2: YOUR BUDGET

While this is not my area of expertise, I'd be remiss if I didn't mention the importance of considering your budget before the next steps.

Today's village is going to come with a price tag for some of the important things you decide your family needs. Mapping out what your budget can handle will help you decide what's needed in your village. It'll also help you determine what areas you can save money on and what you want to save up for.

STEP 3: ENLIST THE PROFESSIONALS

Childcare

Embarking on the journey to finding proper childcare services that fit your family's needs is an overwhelming, stressful-ass task that unfortunately has to be done. Do we agree?

Let's break your choices down from a professional's perspective to help you understand the available choices and the realistic possibilities of them being right for your family.

Childcare facilities are amazing! As a childcare business owner, I highly recommend finding a great facility you and your children will love. But the hard truth about childcare facilities is there is a cap on how many children each facility can hold per age group and per classroom. Typically, parents are unaware of this fact and seemingly heartbroken when they're told either space is not available, or there's a waiting list for that age group or classroom. I always suggest to our prospective families to investigate alternative care while they wait for their ideal location to become available. Here are some other options to support your family's needs for childcare.

Family Daycare Homes

These are smaller daycare programs located in the childcare provider's home. These are a great place to start, especially for younger children in need of full-time or part-time childcare. I started my family daycare—A Giants Preschool—in 2012 and had the privilege of helping many families meet their childcare needs as they returned to work, grew their families, started businesses, and so much more. Added perks of family daycare homes are they can offer the flexibility some families are searching for. Some have non-traditional hours of care available for night and evening workers and tend to have smaller groups of children with the same childcare providers. The biggest myth concerning family daycare homes is that they're not licensed or regulated like commercial childcare facilities and don't offer children educational programs. This is not true for all daycare homes. Depending on the state, a childcare provider must be licensed to operate a childcare home if they care for more than three children who are not their own. Some states require a license for one child. Please check with your state to understand the requirements before enrolling in a program.

Nannies

This is in-your-home care for your children that is a comfortable and safe space for the children. This comes with added perks of later hours, possible meal prep, laundry, dishes, and pet care while you work. Cameras can be set up to keep things transparent, and homeschooling activities can be planned to make sure that your children learn while being cared for at home. This option could be right for you if you work later hours and need non-traditional care hours such as nights and weekends.

Nanny-share opportunities: This is the same as a nanny but typically part-time and shared with other children. You could offer your home as the headquarters for the nanny to include one or two children close to your child's age to offer the bonus of socialization for your little ones. This can be a perk to a family within the village you're cultivating, or it could be the start of a new member of the village. Choosing to nanny share will offer your children some socialization that may not happen with a regular full-time nanny. This could also lower costs as the family that hosts the nanny share often pays less. If you're not the host, this can still help lower your cost as this is part-time care and shared billing for the nanny. The biggest myth for nanny and nanny-share opportunities is that they are here to take care of your home and the child. Contracts are important to outline the responsibilities and expectations of the nanny.

There are also au pairs, babysitters, and family members as options for caring for children other than traditional childcare.

Cleaners/organizers

Parents, moms especially, bear the responsibility of keeping life as clean and organized as possible to be at least able to function. Adding cleaners to your village will help make life a little smoother for the entire family. Bonus if you can hire a cleaner that also organizes. Ahh-that's the windows of heaven opening for you.

Locating such an angel may take time and tenacity, but they're out there.

Having a cleaner come for the entire house is the dream! But to keep costs low, you could hire a cleaner for specific areas of your home, such as the bathrooms and kitchen. Or maybe enlist a laundry service-there's an app for that! This can help you manage the laundry, helping to keep things functionally clean and tidy.

Some nannies work spare hours as house cleaners or organizers and may do laundry. Thinking outside of the box to get the jobs done cost-effectively!

Food shopping/meal prep

Having help to grocery shop can help you get the things you need while simultaneously working on other things. This has been extremely helpful while living a busy life post-COVID. Using Instacart or a similar platform can save you an immense amount of time, effort, and energy. But it may cost you a little money.

Platforms as such are best used with a membership. Having a membership lowers fees for you and allows you to still take advantage of the time and energy-saving perks.

But meal prep is a different story. Finding a reputable company that can feed your family healthy, affordable meals is a larger task. Simply because of food allergies, eating habits, and types, you will need to find a place that makes or prepares what you like to eat. Again, they are out there. It may take time to locate, try, and keep them and their quality services.

Other services can be added to your village depending on your family's needs and budget.

As a pillar in a couple of villages myself and the cultivator of my own village, having help helps! Not doing this all alone, not needing to be in twelve places at one time, and knowing there's someone who can step in when I need them to allows me more time to breathe, to work to build my dreams, and to be in control of life and my family's needs.

The village is still needed even if we must create the village ourselves.

We recognize that the same steps to cultivate a village can pose significant obstacles. Therefore, we have provided resources to help you get started.

Resources to build your village:

- care.com Here, you can find childcare, nanny, pet, and elderly care.
- angieslist.com Great for handymen, house cleaners, and yard care services.
- instacart.com Grocery shopping and food delivery services
- doordash.com Food and more delivery service
- sittercity.com Find babysitters, nannies, or tutoring services.
- blueapron.com Meal prep delivery service
- hellofresh.com Meal prep delivery service

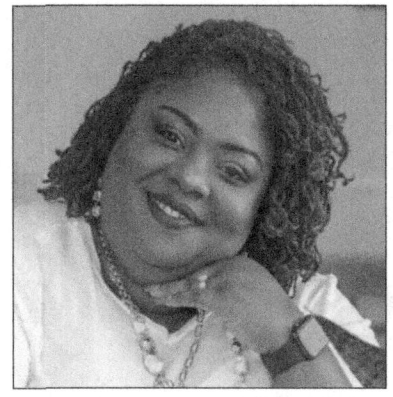

Tomika Robertson is the Owner and Director of A Giants Preschool and A Giants Early Learning Center located in Edgewater, Maryland.

Born and raised in the Washington DC area, Tomika embarked on her childcare career right after high school, starting as an Assistant Teacher in the Infant Program, gaining her certifications to teach Preschool, pre-K 3 teacher, and pre-K 4 in the DC, Maryland Metro area.

Early Childhood Education is my passion.

If you are in the Edgewater, Maryland area and need amazing childcare, look up A Giants Preschool and A Giants Early Learning Center

www.agiantspreschool.com

www.Facebook.com/agiantselc

www.facebook.com/agiants.preschool

CHAPTER 12

A Positive Spin on Parenting

HOW TO KEEP THE VIBE HIGH EVEN IN YOUR FRUSTRATING MOMENTS

Aubrey Edwards, CEO, Bright Beginning Children's Learning Center

MY STORY

My eight-year-old self is sleeping soundly in my bed, dreaming of pitching at my next softball game and bike rides to the park with friends.

"Knock, knock," as my mother opened my bedroom door. "It's time to wake up; it's chore day!"

"Ugh, Mom! It's too early in the morning!"

"You better not make me come in here again!" She says as she heads out to the kitchen.

Sitting up in my bed on a Saturday, rubbing my eyes, stretching, and yawning: *Why do I have the mother that makes us get up every Saturday morning to clean?!*

There we were, my mother, sister, and I, cleaning the house from top to bottom while my dad was outside doing dad stuff, like cutting grass, raking leaves, sorting his tools, or in the shed.

We woke up every Saturday morning to clean our house from childhood until we moved out.

Sometimes my sister and I had to do the chores together, like picking up dog poop, and, dear God, if you were the one holding the bag and the other one accidentally got poop on your fingers! Oh, the screams! We had an attitude, not with each other, but about the fact we had to do this at the crack of dawn or any time for that matter.

As a kid and even in my late teens, I never understood why my mom was so strict about keeping our home in order.

The time came when my family was moving out of our childhood home leaving the state of Maryland and headed for West Virginia. The idea of living in the mountains where your neighbor was miles away and you had to travel thirty minutes for milk was not my cup of tea.

I met with my boss and told her how I didn't want to leave. I loved where I lived, I loved where I worked, and the thought of leaving gave me a ball of stress in my stomach the size of a bowling ball. She mentioned, "My brother just moved to Maryland," she said, "He doesn't like where he's currently living and wants to find a nicer place."

With her help, we found a place for us that we could move into immediately.

I apprehensively told my parents I was staying. It didn't go over well with my mom, but in time, she came around.

The day came for our move-in. My boss's brother brought what he had, and I brought what I had. I only had my bedroom set and a couch from a relative who was getting ready to donate it.

I jokingly said to myself, even though I was serious, "I can't believe I have to buy my own Q-Tips, wrapping paper, and all the things?! Who knew?" I remember having to return hand towels and bathmats because I was short on money and needed food. Living on your own was a lot harder than I ever expected.

I quickly started to realize the importance of keeping a clean place, budgeting your money, and buying only what was needed. In those moments, I remember my mom always saying, "Take care of the things you have because that's all you have!"

Months went by, and we decided to get a third roommate to help cut the costs of living on our own. I moved to the dining room, and she had the Primary bedroom.

We knew nothing about her; back in those days, you found a roommate on Craigslist. Thank goodness she wasn't a murderer, but it ended up being far worse than that. She came with ferrets—smelly, stinky, messy weasels.

It was horrible!

As our year ended in our apartment, I decided I wouldn't renew and moved in with a close friend. The rent would be cheaper; I would no longer live in a dining room, and I'd known her and her husband for years.

Over the next almost decade, I moved in and out of places and spaces until it was time to find my own place since I had a baby.

I was a single mom with a dysfunctional mess, but I had a beautiful baby boy.

With the help of friends, we found a basement apartment off Craigslist. These renters could have been murderers, too, but I took my chances because I was going to be homeless.

For the next two years, I made this basement apartment a home for me and my son. Remembering all those times my mom made me wake up when the sun would rise to clean, in these times, I understood why.

Let me dedicate one morning a week to deep cleaning.

I took what my mom said when I was a kid about our home and applied it to my new little home because that's all I had. I knew I better take care of it.

I would wake up every Saturday morning to enjoy my coffee on my couch, then would quickly start to clean. I got it out of the way to enjoy and savor the rest of our weekend and new week with a clean space for my mind, body, and soul.

I love the quote, "Clutter doesn't just occupy the house in which you live, it occupies your mind," by Avina Celeste.

As time went on, my son's father and I started our relationship again, and we moved into a bigger apartment. I took my routine and mindset into this new space.

It had been a long time since I had to share space with people (and those God-awful ferrets); it was a whole new ball game again!

Living with others who do not have the same routine and mindset is…how do I put this nicely? Challenging!

I'll skip to the part where it didn't work out, and I was on my own as a single mother to two boys.

For me to *keep calm and carry on,* I'm someone who must have a clutter-free life in my home, work, car, mind, and all that I do. Clutter-free to me means that I'm organized, everything has its place, and I know what I'm doing.

As a single mother, I took what I learned from my mom and my experiences through adulthood and into motherhood and found what works for me, my boys, and our home when it comes to staying organized, creating a consistent routine, and all the ways to keep my sanity.

Let me break it down for you!

I have 11 calendars on my Google Calendar, which includes seven for work and four for personal events. I also have a holiday calendar and a task list. If you're the type of gal like me who needs to cross each item off your to-do list, the task list is perfect for you! Once you complete each item, you just click "complete," and it's now off your plate (and calendar). This is what keeps me organized and free of night sweats and panic attacks.

Every night, I have a routine that I follow; I check the Google calendar for any special days or upcoming events for myself and my kids. If they have pajama day, I don't want them to miss out. If I signed up to bring snacks for my kids' school, I sort it out the night before. As I check all that there is for the next day, I'm also looking at the weather app. My oldest son runs hot; if it's a slightly warmer day and he's in fleece sweatpants and a sweater, he will be miserable at school all day.

I pick out their clothes and lay them nicely on our dining room table, and then I grab their backpacks and put them next to the clothes. Then off to the kitchen to make their lunches and stick them in the fridge with their water bottles.

I do as much as I can the night before because I've learned the hard way that if you do these things in the morning, you're rushing around with little to no patience and probably using a few curse words until you're finally out the door.

Other things that keep me organized are the alarms set on my phone. Yes, I have them to wake up to in the morning, but also for vitamins, medicine, and any other reminders, like "Don't forget to bring my kids' bike to school for Bike Day when we leave." If we're walking out the door at 7:30, I have the alarm set with a bike emoji at 7:25.

It's helpful that my youngest son goes to the school I work for, so I'm more up-to-date on what's happening at his school versus my oldest son's school, where they are still sending paper reminders. Those papers sometimes come home or get stuffed in his locker, and I don't see them for months. My oldest son is working on how to be organized. He'll get there—one day.

I've talked a lot about my work in my story, as it's a big part of my life. I'll never understand why people rate work or family as more important. You can't put them in the same category. You must find a balance. Work is what provides for my family and is something I'm very passionate about.

I've worked in childcare for almost twenty-four years, working my way up from being a Teacher Assistant for four of those years, a Lead Teacher for eight years, and a Director for eight years. Four years ago, I moved into the Executive Director position to work alongside the owner, AliceAnne (You'll read about her in this book. She's amazing!).

During the time I moved into my new role, we shifted our preschool into a Positive Preschool. What that means is that currently, four of our administrators and teachers have completed the Positive Education Certification through The Center for Positive Education and apply all that was learned into the classrooms, with the children as well as the staff and families.

The definition of Positive Psychology is the scientific study of strengths that enable individuals and communities to thrive. It was founded on the belief that people want to lead meaningful and fulfilling lives, cultivate what is best within themselves, and enhance their experiences of love, work, and play. (www.authentichappiness.sas.upenn.edu)

Every month, the four of us have a meeting to focus on a topic. Some of the topics include mindset, strengths, kindness, connection, and rituals/routine. Some activities have included affirmations, breath work, yoga poses, decorating kindness rocks and putting them in our playground or neighborhood, donating to charities, and having a successful routine at home. We also incorporate books into the classrooms that relate to the topics, activities to do at home with families and friends, as well as ice breakers with our team.

Along with staying organized and having a clean space, Positive Psychology is something I've incorporated into my life with my boys and our home.

THE TOOL

Here are some tips and tools on how I went from surviving to thriving!

1. HAVE A CONSISTENT ROUTINE

a. When there is a routine with children, there are fewer tears and tantrums. This includes bedtime at night and waking up in the morning. When they know what to expect each day they're more confident and secure and less stressed. Obviously, things come up, like doctor's appointments, vacations, etc., but overall, there needs to be consistency. Create a visual schedule for your children that can be placed in their bedroom or in an area they can see at eye level. They can check it off or move an arrow to the next time slot.

2. SLEEP IS IMPORTANT

a. Speaking of bedtime routines, getting good sleep is vital for children. Set a regular bedtime and stick to it. My boys' nighttime routine consists of bath or shower time, vitamins, a snack, a little bit of water, and then book time. This typically takes about an hour and a half to two hours in total. Once everyone is down and out, I'm usually right behind them, as it's vital for parents to get good sleep as well!

3. SHIFT YOUR MINDSET

a. Having a growth mindset means that you are capable of improvement and change. Have you ever been around someone who is always negative? They suck you dry. I love the quote, "Attitudes are contagious; is yours worth catching?" I've posted this quote on our private work Facebook page several times because it's true. Working with or parenting children is hard; when your spouse or co-worker is being a Negative Nancy, it affects you and the people around you, meaning the children. "Nancy, can you walk away and take some breaths, give yourself a moment, and then come back? That would be great." When there's downtime, chat with each other and, while being mindful, share that when they're being negative, it's a domino effect, and it's hard to get through a day like that. Give them the space and grace when they're feeling any sort of way and validate their feelings. This all needs to be at an appropriate time.

b. Add affirmations, quotes, and mantras to your bathroom mirror or the inside of your closet to remind yourself every morning; this will help shift your mindset and set you up for the day.

4. USE YOUR STRENGTHS

a. Have you ever been to an interview, and they ask you what you do well in, and it takes you a minute to think about the answer? We're so programmed to focus on what we don't excel in, and we also tend to make ourselves feel better by finding what others don't excel in either. Instead of focusing on shortcomings, let's focus on what we all do well! There's an assessment that we use called the Character's Strengths Assessment through https://www.viacharacter.org/. There is even a children's assessment as well! This assessment will show you your 24 strengths. Yep, we have 24 strengths in our toolbox. While it states to focus on the top five, think of the other 19 as backup. Going back to the toolbox analogy, if my strengths are in honesty, perseverance, leadership, fairness, and humor, and I have a friend or my child crying on my shoulder that life or homework is hard, I'm not going to use honesty or humor in this situation; I'm going to dig down deep in my toolbox and look for my other strengths to help in this situation. The top five give yourself and others a preview of what you excel in. If they want honest feedback, I'm your girl. If they want someone to show up as a leader who won't give up, come to me. But if you're looking for zest, it'll always be at the bottom. I would have to dig way down deep to find a little zest. This is a fun assessment that you can do with family, friends, and co-workers.

5. TRY TO ELIMINATE THE STRESSORS

a. As I said before, when there is consistency and a routine, people thrive. Will there be obstacles and things popping up that we can't control? Absolutely! Here are some suggestions that can help your children and even yourself.

b. Along with getting good sleep, move your body, even if it's just for fifteen minutes a day. Walk around your neighborhood, get the bikes out, or kick the ball in your backyard. Exercise is one of the best ways to help reduce stress.

c. Find your tribe, whether it's girlfriends, your spouse, or work friends. Healthy relationships are important for our well-being.

d. Eating a balanced and varied diet, too. Our brain is maintained by the food we eat.

6. CHOOSE YOUR BATTLES

a. Speaking of food, we grew up in times when families only served one meal, and you didn't get up until your plate was clear. Canned mixed vegetables were the death of me! My children will get a variety of protein, fruit, vegetables, and starches on their plates. If they don't eat all of it, it's because I know they're full. My children will refuse certain foods; one will eat all the vegetables while the other only likes fruits. You must do what's best for you and your children. Just continue putting it on their plate. Over time, taste buds change, and they may try it and like it. Also, my children love to help me cook and bake. Get your children involved in the cooking process; they are more likely to try what they make!

7. SELF-CARE ISN'T SELFISH

a. As a parent, especially a single one, you can do a lot of things, but you can't do all the things! Give yourself a break. If you can schedule a self-care day once a month, whether that's getting your nails done, a massage, or lunch with friends, that's great! Self-care is also having some alone time, watching a movie, reading a book, or finding a hobby. Find what you like and what's best for you, and schedule it!

8. PRESENCE OVER PRESENTS

a. A couple of years ago, I shifted from spending tons of money on gifts and parties (adding a sprinkle of stress for the upcoming holidays and birthdays) and chose to take my boys on adventures! My boys and I love going to new places, and this helps build a connection with each other, all while making memories. I rotate between free to low costs and one to two bigger experiences, like the beach or Dutch Wonderland and Cartoon Network Hotel. I map out the entire year to see how to properly budget for these adventures. During the holiday months, I look for free to low-cost places. Check out Color Burst Park in Columbia and Watkins Park in Upper Marlboro, or even Anne Arundel County Park and Rec. Lots of free to low-cost activities that are so fun for little ones!

All of these things didn't happen overnight, and it has taken me a while to stick to it; however, with consistency, it was a smooth transition. My goal for shifting to having a consistent routine and staying organized was to eliminate the feeling of chaos and stress in my life as well as my boys' lives. My children and I deserve a calm morning for a productive and successful day at school, work, and all that we do. I encourage you to find the best routine for you and your family, as well as add Positive Psychology into your every day.

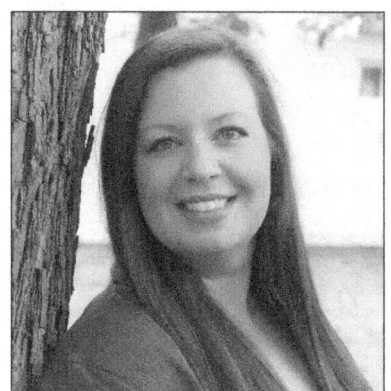

Aubrey Edwards is the CEO of Bright Beginning Children's Learning Center. BBCLC has two convenient locations in Anne Arundel County for ages 2-5 (Crownsville #130684 and Glen Burnie # 160256). She is consistently completing professional development hours and is currently taking online courses at Anne Arundel Community College. Aubrey has earned her Teacher Certification, Positive Education Certification, Coaching & Mentoring Certification, and Director of Operations Certification. She started with BBCLC when they first opened their doors in September of 2004 and has a total of 24 years of experience working in Early Education. Over the years, she was a Pre-K Assistant and Teacher as well as a Site Director, and currently the Executive Director.

Aubrey has always been passionate about working with children and making a difference in every child's life that walks through BBCLC's doors. Her mission has always been to create a safe, nurturing, and fun environment for all children to learn and grow.

She is also very passionate about training, supporting, and helping all staff to gain as much knowledge when it comes to BBCLC's Mission and Vision and see that it gets carried through.

Aubrey currently resides in Glen Burnie, Maryland, with her two boys, Cruz (age 9) and Enzo (age 2). They love trying new experiences, spending as much time outside, and going out to eat.

For more information on Positive Psychology, as well as tips and tools for every day, be sure to check out our blogs! https://bright-beginning.com/blog/

For more information on Bright Beginning Children's Learning Center, you can follow us

Website: www.bright-beginning.com

Facebook: https://www.facebook.com/bright.beginning867

Instagram: @bbclc

My contact information:

a.edwards@bright-beginning.com

CHAPTER 13

How to Calm Your Nervous System in 60 Seconds

AN ANYTIME BREATH TOOL FOR OVERWHELM

Trish Brewer, Certified Breathwork Coach

MY STORY

I used to feel guilty all the time! Guilty if I ate too much. Guilty if I go out with my girlfriends. Guilty for not making a home-cooked meal every day. Guilty for being a working mom. I was a burned-out and overwhelmed mom, and it landed me in the hospital for a week.

Self-care, rest, and relaxation don't come easy for many of us, myself included. The model I inherited was one of relentless work and self-sacrifice, particularly for the sake of family.

Juggling multiple roles—mother, wife, chef, homemaker, daughter, employee, sibling, friend—while striving for perfection in maintaining a pristine home, preparing homemade meals, and meeting societal standards is an exhausting and relentless cycle.

Overwhelm intensifies mom guilt, and mom guilt contributes to overwhelm. Round and round we go. I know it well; I was stuck in the merry-go-round of it. I can't pinpoint when exactly this guilt showed up in my life, but it is deeply embedded in my psyche and body.

The first-born child of lower-middle-class Italian Catholic immigrants, I felt guilt at every "wrong" turn. Whether it was the time I lied in the confessional booth at seven years old or when I moved away from home at eighteen while my dad was terminally ill, both left an imprint on my consciousness. One consisted of Catholic guilt condemning me to Hell, and the other the Italian guilt of abandoning my family. The expectations were high, whether self-imposed or not, and I came to epitomize "Catholic guilt." No one is to blame here; it was just the circumstances.

But even Catholic guilt can't equate to working mom guilt; it's the worst! You're damned if you do and damned if you don't. You can never seem to get the balance quite right; at least, I can't. Some ball is eventually going to be dropped, and the ensuing guilt is practically unavoidable, not to mention the overwhelm along the way.

Did I pump enough breast milk?

What if he runs out and gets hungry?

Did I pack enough diapers?

Where am I going to pump?

What will my co-workers think about how much time I'm taking to do so?

What am I going to wear?

Am I a bad mom for leaving him to go to work?

Breathe, Trish, breathe.

He will be okay.

These were the thoughts echoing through my head as I paced between the kitchen, opening the freezer and counting the bags of frozen breast milk for the fifth time, then to the baby's room, checking the diaper bag again to make sure there were enough diapers, then to the bedroom closet to check the outfits I selected, all with baby in tow wondering how could I leave this precious bundle. Life changed twelve weeks ago and was about to change again as I shifted from a new mom to a working mom.

I had all intentions of breastfeeding my child for his first year. It's what a good mother does. It was the best and most natural form of nourishment you could provide, so I believed. Then, the day came when I no longer produced enough breastmilk to sustain him. I went back to work full-time, and it was challenging to pump at regular intervals. I'm not sure I'll ever forget the guilt and shame overwhelming me the first time I had to supplement his feedings with formula.

He didn't bring lunch with him today. Is it okay if we give him mac-n-cheese? Of course! Oh, darn, we must have left lunch at home. Thank you! (Insert feelings of guilt and shame.)

Breathe, Trish, breathe.

You are only human. We all make mistakes.

He will be okay.

* * *

Mom, I need a dish for the Spanish Heritage Celebration tomorrow.

Really!? And you're telling me now? At 5 pm, when I have a client at 6 pm.

I forgot.

(Insert feelings of overwhelm.)

Breathe, Trish, breathe.

You got this. He will be okay if the dish is not perfect.

* * *

Eventually, the culmination of years of burnout, the overwhelm of working mom guilt, unrealistic expectations, juggling multiple roles and responsibilities, and the lack of self-care and boundaries landed me in the hospital for a week with excruciating abdominal pains. After a series of extensive tests and scans, the medical team concluded I was grappling with an inexplicable bacterial infection in my gastrointestinal tract, triggering a severe bout of acute pancreatitis.

This medical emergency knocked me out of my comfort zone and forced a change in my lifestyle. I could no longer ignore my own needs. I realized to take care of the ones I loved I'd have to start with myself. And so began my recovery to heal not just my body but all of me, finally recognizing the connection of the body/mind/spirit. I started to meditate daily and journal my thoughts and feelings. I went to therapy and received Reiki and acupuncture.

Then, two years later, on a June afternoon in Stratton, Vermont, breathwork found me. An unfolding began as deep layers of stored trauma surfaced. From there, the healing within began and rippled outward. More moved through me in those forty-five minutes than in a lifetime. And I had been doing "the work." I even co-led a women's group centered around spiritual empowerment. But breathwork cracked me wide open! It was the healing modality calling me home.

My body trembled and cramped as the energy coursed through it. Tears flowed as the trauma of old wounds came to the surface and then left. I felt the warm embrace of my Nona Santina as she put my heart and mind at ease through it all. I saw the face of my dad come to me, filling me with strength. It was sad, it was gut-wrenching, and it was beautiful all at once. It left me longing for more. I knew I had just barely scraped the surface of my healing.

Throughout the summer, I continued to peel back the layers through many virtual sessions. By the end of the summer, I had completed my first level of breathwork training, and by the end of the following summer, the first of my certifications. To say breathwork has changed the trajectory of my life is an understatement. I liken it to more of a remembering. I returned from Vermont with purpose. It gave me a peace I didn't know before.

Breathwork was the breakthrough for me. It marked the next level of energy work, unveiling a layer of my life and granting me profound clarity and peace about what was truly essential. I had to redefine what the "good mother" looked like.

Challenging cultural narratives around motherhood for me looked like splitting household chores and childcare with my husband, making time for a monthly book club, going away for an annual weekend retreat, and letting go of the notion the house had to be neat and clean 24/7. In my Italian home, I grew up with women being responsible for everything inside the house (including child rearing) and men being responsible for the outside of the house, except for the garden, which we all tended to.

In the beginning, I asked myself:

Am I a bad mother because I'm choosing to go to book club with my girlfriends instead of staying home with my family?

Am I a bad mom because I'm going away for a weekend retreat, leaving my child and husband to fend for themselves?

Am I being selfish? I never saw my mom do these things.

I had to be okay with the perceived imperfections of not keeping a clean home and eating out on occasion. Over time, I slowly embraced my individuality in motherhood, shifting my perspective out of the vicious cycle of mom guilt and overwhelm. It was, and still is, a daily practice. For me, it's setting aside time before the morning bustle starts for a five-minute breath practice, a five-minute meditation, and five minutes of journaling.

I've learned a good mother:

- Isn't one who does it all but instead asks for help.
- Tends to her own needs, especially in moments of overwhelm.
- Celebrates her imperfections.
- Becomes comfortable with saying "I'm sorry," to her children.

I've learned there is no true definition of a "good mother" as we continue to redefine the role of motherhood, and each of us is making it our own.

I can't lie; the working mom guilt creeps its way back in from time to time. Usually, it's when the ball drops, and inevitably, it does because we're all human, and perfection, like control, is an illusion. Or when a passive-aggressive comment is made by another parent or teacher, or when I'm questioned by a family member because I took a weekend away to restore my mind/body/soul.

There will always be someone around to criticize or offer an opinion, whether you ask them to or not. On the good days, it rolls off my back with ease, and on the worst days, it triggers the inner child, bringing me back to where it all began.

In those moments, my breath is the most powerful tool in my toolbox. I use it to help regulate my nervous system in moments of overwhelm, crisis, panic, anxiety, etc. I use it to move through old patterns, stories, and misbeliefs accumulated in my body.

Breath is our life force. It was the first thing we did when we came into this world and the last thing we will do before we leave this Earth. Yet so many of us move through the day without any regard for it, without any thought as to its strength or power, taking it for granted, without really knowing how to breathe properly. Instead, most take shallow breaths from their chest. When we breathe deeply from our diaphragm, think belly rise and fall, we can shift out of living "wired and tired."

My purpose is to teach others the power their breath holds and how they can use it to release emotional and mental blocks in their bodies as well as calm and center their nervous system.

As mothers, we have the innate ability to help our children and our communities just by helping ourselves first. Our children learn through what we model for them. Imagine being able to shift from overwhelmed mom to grounded mom in 60 seconds with a built-in tool! Then imagine teaching your kids the same!

THE TOOL

So often, we're told to pause and take a breath, but we're not taught how or why. It is my commitment to teach you both.

I've found the simplest and most effective breath tool for coming back to yourself in a moment of overwhelm, or any big feelings, really, is **balance breathing**. This equal inhale and equal exhale breath technique through the nose soothes the nervous system.

4:4 Balance Breathing Exercise

Step 1: Take a comfortable seated position. Place one hand over your belly and one hand over your chest. Close your eyes or find a soft gaze on a place in your space. Make sure your chin is parallel to the floor, and relax your belly, face, and shoulders. (This step is ideal but not necessary. If you're in the moment or on the go, adjust to the situation. But do try to relax your belly, face, and shoulders.)

Step 2: Inhale through the nose for a count of four, feeling the belly rise and expand with each inhale.

Step 3: Exhale through the nose for a count of four, feeling the belly collapse back towards the spine with each exhale.

Step 4: Repeat nine more times.

This straightforward breathing exercise stimulates the parasympathetic nervous system, commonly referred to as "rest and digest." This activation works to decrease your heart rate and induce relaxation in your internal organs, guiding you to a state of tranquility and alleviating feelings of anxiety and stress.

Use this breath technique anytime to calm and center yourself.

When and where to use this technique

In the beginning, it's good to practice this technique daily. Set a reminder on your phone if you need to. Do it before you get out of bed in the morning; do it right before lunch (my favorite time). But make it a priority so this technique becomes second nature.

Because you are inhaling and exhaling through your nose, no one even knows you're doing it! So, you can practice this breath technique anywhere!

Just a Few Examples:
- In line at the grocery store while your child is having a complete meltdown.
- In the car at a stop light (don't close your eyes) when the kids are fighting in the back seat.
- When you walk into the house to a pile of dishes in the sink and feel your heart begin to race.

- When you're trying to get the kiddo(s) down for a nap, and your partner calls to add something to your to-do list.
- When the work presentation is in five minutes and daycare calls because your child just threw up.

History

The 4:4 balance breath technique, adapted from Stephen Eliott's Coherent Breathing, focuses on reducing the number of breaths per minute to induce mental relaxation and regulate the nervous system. Although developed in the early 2000s, the practice of controlling one's breath, known as pranayama, has been a cornerstone of yoga for millennia.

Pranayama is the Sanskrit term for yoga breathing. It combines "prana" (life force) with "yama" (extension or control), encapsulating the essence of breath regulation. Essentially, Pranayama can be defined as "the regulation and expansion of life energy through breath."

The roots of breathing practices extend back to pre-common era (CE) times, documented in sacred texts such as the Upanishads, Bhagavad Gita, Yoga Sutras, and Hathapradipika. These practices were traditionally associated with higher states of consciousness, mysticism, self-awareness, and transcendence, with a belief that slowing the breath correlated with an extended lifespan.

In the 1900s, breathing practices became integral to various yoga styles, influencing contemporary classes worldwide. As we entered the 2000s, these practices gained popularity beyond the realm of yoga, often pursued for singular benefits, detached from the broader context of holistic well-being.

Why does breathing help so much?

Here's an abbreviated version of the science behind the why.

There are two branches of the autonomic nervous system: sympathetic (fight and flight) and parasympathetic (rest and digest). A balanced nervous system is our goal.

The autonomic nervous system controls the heart rate, digestion, respiratory rate, pupillary response, urination, and sexual arousal.

When our nervous system is in a **parasympathetic (rest & digest)** state, the body's response is an increase in blood flow to the stomach and GI tract, stimulation of peristalsis, urination, and salivary glands, a decrease in the heart rate, pupil normalization for shorter-range vision, and sexual arousal.

When our nervous system is in a **sympathetic (fight or flight)** state, our digestion and elimination stop, blood goes to muscles and lungs as much as 12 times more, epinephrine (adrenaline) goes up, heart rate increases, pupils dilate for better long-distance vision, and we reach sexual orgasm.

The vagus nerve is the tenth cranial nerve and the longest of the autonomic nervous system. It's technically a pair of nerves but referred to as singular. It's a "Vagabond" nerve, meaning it has little branches that go everywhere.

Deep breathing stimulates the vagus nerve, which is largely responsible for the parasympathetic response (rest and digest). The vagus nerve controls the heart, lungs, and digestive tract, and it runs through an opening in the diaphragm. Breathing, singing, humming, and chanting all promote vagal tone and enable the body to self-soothe.

A Few Benefits of Breathwork:
- Reduces stress, anxiety, and depression.
- Balances mood/energy.
- Increases mental focus.
- Improves sleep.
- Boosts digestion.
- Resets the nervous system.

Lessens Anxiety, Depression, and Stress - Deep breathing activates the parasympathetic nervous system, taking us out of "fight and flight." This also slows down the heart rate and lowers blood pressure, bringing us to a place of tranquility and reducing those feelings of anxiety and stress.

Aids in Sleep and Improves Digestion - Deep breathing techniques with longer exhales help to calm our nervous system and reduce overstimulation negatively impacting our sleep. In addition, this reduces the heart rate, simultaneously increasing the blood flow to the stomach and GI tract.

Increases Self-Awareness - Breathwork allows you to move out of the intellect of your mind and get into your body, allowing you to deeply connect with yourself. Creating better emotional intelligence and promoting clarity in thought, communication, and action.

Breath Tools vs Breathwork

Breathwork is a very popular and powerful tool getting lots of hype today. Know the difference between breath tools and breathwork (healing).

Breath Tools are breath techniques used at the moment and can be incorporated into daily practice for a healthier, less stressful life.

Examples: Box Breath, Alternate Nostril Breathing, 4:7:8 relaxing breath, Wim Hoff, and Breath of Fire.

Breathwork (Healing) is a deeper, more sacred, and spiritual practice. It's an active, efficient, and effective technique that allows you to disconnect from the thinking mind and enter a heightened state of consciousness.

Examples: Rebirthing by Leonard Orr, Holotropic by Christina Grof and Stanislav Grof, and Breathwork by David Elliott.

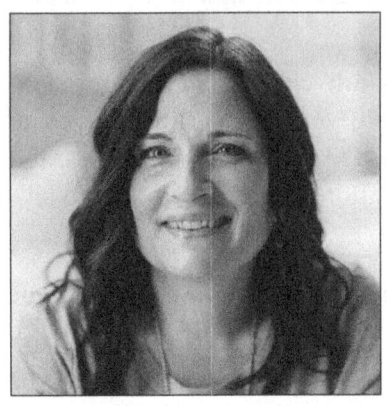

Trish Brewer is a certified trauma-informed breathwork coach, Reiki Master Teacher, and intuitive guide who'll be your guide back to your whole self. Whether you're overwhelmed, unable to cope with life's challenges, or find yourself in a period of transition, she's there to create a nurturing and compassionate space to begin healing. She believes when we allow ourselves to be supported, we expedite our healing and self-discovery.

As an intuitive guide, Trish employs a trauma-aware approach, utilizing the transformative elements of breathwork, processing work, and Reiki to guide individuals back to their complete selves. Her sessions are sensitively designed to anticipate the messy and unexpected aspects of the healing process, acknowledging both the light and the dark and witnessing the beauty along the way.

Trish earned her Breath Coach Certification from Yoga Teachers College, studied under David Elliot, a Breathwork pioneer, received her Usui/Holy Fire® Reiki training through Divine Tri Source, and completed her trauma training with the NeuroAffective Relational Model (NARM) Training Institute, and continues her work today with Gwen Dittmar. She sees herself as a lifelong student.

Trish believes healing oneself ripples outward and is committed to donating a meaningful percentage of her time and proceeds to national and community charities, including the National Ovarian Cancer Coalition, Black Girls Breathing, and the May-B Foundation.

She resides in southern Maryland with her son, husband, and rescue dog. Her stepdaughter, a market research analyst and artist, lives in Newport, RI.

Connect with Trish

Email: trish@trishbrewer.com

Website: https://www.trishbrewer.com/

Instagram: https://www.instagram.com/trishbrewerbreathwork/

Facebook: https://www.facebook.com/trishdbrewerbreathwork/

LinkedIn: https://www.linkedin.com/in/trish-brewer-5b467025/

Free Resources

Link to 4:4 Balance Breath Video:

https://youtu.be/V-nuNoziNQo?si=aBtSPxwd37TyQiZZ

Link to 4:4 Balance Breath Video for Kids:

https://youtu.be/8NRS3MAMpBU?si=wiyEgdIQ38XgPOly

CHAPTER 14

A Nourishing Balance

FEEL GOOD FEEDING BABY
AND FUELING YOUR BODY

Beth Conlon, PhD, RDN

MY STORY

The Truth About Postpartum Nutrition

As a Registered Dietitian Nutritionist, I assumed that feeding my newborn and bouncing back after having a baby would be a walk in the park. I envisioned an idyllic postpartum experience:

- Lovingly nursing my sweet baby while gently rocking in a cozy chair.
- Pumping ounces of breast milk for storage with ease.
- Eating "perfect" or "clean" foods that would provide optimal nourishment to both my baby and myself.
- Juggling motherhood, work, and personal time with grace.
- Being back in my pre-pregnancy jeans within weeks of giving birth.
- Enjoying plenty of sleep as my baby peacefully rested with scheduled feeding times.
- Maintaining a calm and put-together household despite the addition of a new family member.

- Having enough time and energy to keep up with regular exercise.
- Meeting other mom friends for joyful and relaxing walks in the park.

I quickly learned reality was far from that picture-perfect scenario. The first few months postpartum were a blur of sleepless nights, constant diaper changes, and trying to figure out how to keep a tiny human alive.

I will never forget the time when my first child was just three weeks old. Exhausted and barely awake, I stumbled out of bed yet again in the middle of the night. "I can't do this," I mumbled to myself. My husband, half-asleep, stirred and asked me what was wrong. With weary eyes, I replied, "The baby just won't sleep at all. I don't know what he needs." Determined, I rose from the bed to attend to our newborn, trying various methods to lull him back to sleep. As the hours passed and the sun began to rise, I silently acknowledged that this was our new reality.

It turns out that he wasn't getting full feedings. His latch was painful, and I was struggling with breastfeeding. I was doing a combination of nursing, pumping, and supplementing with formula. Inside, I felt like a complete failure because my milk supply wasn't meeting my baby's needs. To top it off, I was so focused on nourishing my newborn that I neglected to take care of myself. That weight did not melt off.

It wasn't until I reached out to other moms for support and advice that I realized I wasn't alone. My lactation consultant had a private Facebook community that was a lifesaver. I connected with other moms who had similar struggles and learned that what I was experiencing was common. They offered encouragement, reminding me that I was doing the best I could for my baby.

I learned that countless mothers had similar difficulties navigating motherhood and found their own well-being went out the window while caring for their little ones. As new mothers, we often feel immense pressure to be perfect. To have it all together and effortlessly handle the demands of motherhood. But the truth is, it's a struggle. And that's NORMAL. I don't know where these ridiculous standards came from, but we need to let go of them. We need to be kind to ourselves and recognize that it's okay to be filled with joy and love one minute and completely overwhelmed and exhausted the next.

So, to all the new moms out there struggling with their postpartum bodies and feeling overwhelmed—you are amazing. You have brought a precious life into this world, and that makes you a superhero. Take care of yourself, seek support when needed, and know you're not alone. Motherhood is a beautiful, messy, and challenging journey, but it can be filled with so much love and joy if we set realistic expectations for ourselves. Embrace the ups and downs, cherish the moments of snuggles and giggles, and remember to be kind to yourself.

THE TOOL

Feeding Baby: Fed is Best

As I slowly adjusted to my new role as a mom, I realized that what works for one family may not work for another. And I know now that's perfectly fine. In the first few months, feeding your infant can feel like a challenge. It seems like everyone has different advice, and it's easy to get overwhelmed. But healthcare professionals, from lactation consultants and dietitians to pediatricians to researchers, generally agree that there is no one "right" way to feed your baby. You have to find what works best for you and your little one, and at the end of the day, fed is best.

What does 'fed is best' mean? In healthcare, we care about one primary outcome when it comes to nutrition: growth. We want to see that your baby is gaining weight and growing at appropriate rates.

You can achieve this goal by making sure your infant receives the calories and nutrients they need using one of the methods below:

- Breastfeeding
- Bottle-feeding with formula or expressed breastmilk
- Combination feeding (a combination of the above)

Some babies have unique feeding needs and may require alternative methods, such as tube feedings. However, this topic is beyond the scope of this chapter.

Whether it's breastfeeding, formula-feeding, or a combination of both, what matters most is that your baby is getting the nourishment they need. Formulas have made significant improvements in recent years, containing more and more beneficial components found in breastmilk and options for babies with allergies, sensitivities, and other special needs. Breastfeeding, on the other hand, offers benefits such as providing antibodies and nutrition that is optimized for variations in your baby's daily and monthly needs. So remember, whatever feeding method you choose, it's perfectly okay as long as your baby is growing and thriving.

According to the American Academy of Pediatrics (AAP):

- Newborns need to be fed every two to three hours. Older babies may only need to be fed every three to four hours.
- A general guideline is that babies need about two and a half ounces of breast milk or formula per pound of body weight per day.
- It's important to monitor weight gain and diaper output with the help of a pediatrician or lactation consultant to ensure the baby is getting enough nutrition.
- Newborns may initially lose some weight due to water loss but should start gaining weight at an average rate of one ounce per day within the first week.

What feeding method suits you and your baby? Breastfeeding, formula feeding, or combination feeding? Think about the benefits and challenges associated with each.

Reflect on your lifestyle: Consider your daily routine, your work commitments, and your social support system (partner, family, friends). Will any of these feeding methods fit better with your current lifestyle?

Listen to your body: Do you have any health considerations that might affect your ability to breastfeed? If so, how might formula feeding or combination feeding work for you?

Identify your emotions: How do you feel about each method of feeding? Are there any concerns or fears that may arise with one method over the other?

Know that it's natural for mothers to worry about whether their baby is getting enough milk or formula, and it can be overwhelming to try to navigate through the various challenges and obstacles that may arise. Remember to keep an open mind and be gentle with yourself as you reflect on these questions. Feeding your baby is just one aspect of being a parent, and whatever method you choose, remember, there's no one-size-fits-all approach to feeding your baby. The best choice is the one that ensures both your baby's nourishment and your wellbeing. I encourage you to reflect on your personal circumstances and feelings. Each feeding method has its advantages; what matters most is that your baby is fed, loved, and cared for.

There's an old saying that goes, "You can't pour from an empty cup." As a new mom, this saying is truer than ever. While you're busy caring for your newborn, it's important to remember to take care of yourself, too, especially when it comes to nutrition. Postpartum nutrition for both baby and mom is essential, not only for growth and development but also for recuperation and strength.

References:

The Fed is Best Foundation. Fed is Best Guide to Safe Infant Feeding. https://fedisbest.org/wp-content/uploads/2021/03/2020-Edition-Feeding-Plan-for-Baby1.pdf. Updated 2020. Accessed 29 Dec 2023.

"How Often and How Much Should Your Baby Eat?" Healthy Children, American Academy of Pediatrics. www.healthychildren.org/English/ages-stages/baby/feeding-nutrition/Pages/how-often-and-how-much-should-your-baby-eat.aspx. Accessed 29 Dec 2023.

A Non-Diet Approach to Postpartum Nutrition

After my first pregnancy, I wanted so badly to lose my pregnancy weight quickly, but my body wasn't cooperating. I tried restricting calories but ended up constantly hungry and fatigued. Moreover, I worried to myself, "Will reducing calories affect my already low milk supply?"

The postpartum period is a time when your body needs extra care and nourishment for recovery, breastfeeding (if applicable) and energy to care for your little one. But conventional diet and weight-loss-focused methods often add more stress to the postpartum period when you need less! Restrictive dieting practices also don't work well long-term. It wasn't until I embraced a non-diet approach based on The Plate Method that I finally found peace with my body in its current stage of life and nourished myself in a way that supported both me and my baby.

The Plate Method is a compassionate and evidence-based approach that focuses on balance, variety, and moderation without harmful dieting practices. No calorie or macronutrient counting, no apps. This approach can help you achieve and maintain a balanced diet that has many health benefits without being overly restrictive or complicated.

Here's how it works:

The Plate Method is a simple yet versatile tool for planning healthy meals that relies mostly on timing and visualization. In terms of timing, it's recommended to aim for three meals and two to three snacks per day. This looks something like:

- Breakfast
- Mid-morning snack
- Lunch
- Afternoon snack
- Dinner
- Optional evening snack

Day-to-day consistency is key to help regulate postpartum hormones and support metabolic health. If you don't currently have a consistent eating schedule, I suggest picking one area to focus on, such as getting in the habit of eating breakfast within 30-60 minutes of waking up or introducing an afternoon snack.

Now, what to eat at each meal and snack? I love the Plate Method because it emphasizes the visualization of the plate rather than measuring out specific amounts of food. This flexibility allows you to adjust foods and portion sizes based on your hunger and fullness cues without any strict rules or restrictions. And you can take it anywhere from parties and events to vacations.

How To Use The Plate Method

Now let's dive into how you can use the Plate Method to plan and prepare your meals and snacks. The Plate Method divides your plate for meals into three sections: 1/2 the plate for colorful fiber-filled foods (fruits and vegetables), 1/4 the plate for protein, and 1/4 the plate for grains or starchy foods. The goal is to fill your plate with a variety of nutrient-rich foods, promoting well-rounded, balanced meals. For snacks, aim for a combination of fiber-rich foods plus a protein and optional healthy fat.

Here are some examples to help you visualize the Plate Method in action:

- Breakfast: vegetable omelet with whole grain toast and fruit
- Mid-morning snack: Greek yogurt with berries and nuts
- Lunch: grilled chicken salad with quinoa and roasted vegetables
- Afternoon snack: apple slices with nut butter
- Dinner: salmon with brown rice and steamed vegetables, plus a glass of milk
- Evening snack: hummus and pretzels and/or veggie sticks.

This method not only helps you meet your nutrient needs but also lets you be flexible in choosing foods you enjoy. Remember, no single meal or snack has to be perfect. Here's a tip: try the 80/20 rule. Make nourishing choices 80% of the time and give yourself some wiggle room for treats or less nutrient-dense foods the other 20%. This approach can keep you on track with your health goals while still allowing you to enjoy your favorite foods in moderation. Restriction usually backfires and leads to feelings of deprivation and eventual overindulgence. Let's break free from those endless cycles of restrictive and harmful dieting practices!

Proteins

Fill one-quarter of your plate with protein foods. Proteins are essential for repairing tissues and strengthening the immune system.

Here are some protein-rich food ideas:

- Chicken/Turkey
- Lean Beef
- Fish
- Shellfish
- Greek yogurt
- Cottage cheese
- Eggs
- Nuts and seeds
- Nut and seed butters

- Tofu
- Quinoa
- Legumes and Lentils

Carbohydrates/Starches

Fill one-quarter of your plate with carbohydrates or starchy foods. Carbohydrates provide your body with the energy it needs to recover and take care of your newborn.

Here are some carbohydrate-rich food ideas:

- Rice (brown or white)
- Pasta (choose ones higher in fiber and protein)
- Whole grains like quinoa, oats, millet, farro, and barley
- Bread (whole grain or white)
- Crackers
- Buckwheat
- Beans, lentils, and chickpeas
- Sweet potatoes, corn, and peas

When possible, choose whole grains such as brown rice, quinoa, oatmeal, and whole grain bread or pasta, which also pack in beneficial fiber. If you do eat carbohydrates that have little to no fiber, pair it with a source of fiber (like fruits or vegetables) and some protein for a more satiating meal or snack.

Fruits and Vegetables

Half of your plate should be filled with fruits and vegetables, particularly those high in fiber. This aids digestion and prevents constipation, a common postpartum issue. Pile on colorful veggies like spinach, bell peppers, and zucchini and fruits like berries, apples, and oranges—the possibilities are endless! Experiment with different cooking methods, from raw to steamed to baked or sauteed.

Here are some fruit ideas:
- Apples
- Bananas
- Blackberries
- Blueberries
- Grapes
- Oranges
- Peaches
- Pears
- Strawberries
- Watermelon

Here are some vegetable ideas:
- Asparagus
- Bell peppers
- Broccoli
- Brussels sprouts
- Carrots
- Cucumbers
- Green beans
- Spinach or kale
- Tomatoes
- Zucchini

Dairy and Dairy Alternatives

A small serving of dairy or dairy alternatives can offer additional calcium and Vitamin D, crucial for bone health. This could be a glass of milk, a slice of cheese, or a serving of yogurt. You can also opt for fortified soy, almond, or oat milk if you prefer plant-based options that are calcium-fortified.

Here are some dairy ideas:

- Milk
- Cheese
- Yogurt
- Nut and seed milks
- Oat milk
- Soy milk
- Coconut milk
- Vegan cheeses

Healthy Fats

Healthy fats are important for hormone regulation and brain health and help in the absorption of certain vitamins. They also help keep you satiated in between meals and snacks.

Here are some healthy fat ideas:

- Avocados
- Olive oil
- Canola oil
- Flaxseeds and flaxseed oil
- Fatty fish (salmon, mackeral, herring, tuna, sardines)
- Nuts and seeds

Adding healthy fats to meals and snacks can help you stay fuller longer.

Hydration

Staying well-hydrated is equally important as nourishing your body with wholesome food. If you're breastfeeding, your need for fluids increases significantly. Make hydration fun and appealing by investing in a chic water bottle, infusing your water with fruits for a burst of flavor, or opting for flavored waters. A general rule of thumb is to drink half your body weight in ounces of water.

Exercise

Exercise plus nutrition are key components of a healthy postpartum recovery. See chapters 1 and 3 for more information on postpartum exercise.

In summary:

- Fill half of your plate with colorful fruits and vegetables. Aim for a variety of colors, as each color provides different nutrients.
- Choose lean protein sources such as chicken, fish, eggs, or legumes to fill one-quarter of your plate.
- The remaining quarter should be filled with starchy foods like whole grains, potatoes, or sweet potatoes.
- Include healthy fats in your meals and snacks, such as avocados, nuts, flaxseed, chia seeds, and olive oil.
- Experiment with different herbs and spices to add flavor to your dishes.
- Drink plenty of water (aim for one-half of your body weight) throughout the day to stay hydrated and keep your body functioning properly.

The Plate Method is a practical, adaptable approach that promotes a non-diet mentality, fostering a healthier relationship with food. It encourages postpartum women to focus on nutrition rather than restrictions, supporting recovery and overall health. And remember, it's not about perfect execution but gradual, sustainable changes. Each step you take brings you closer to your health and wellness goals for both you and your little one.

I have a wonderful guide you can print to help you navigate thePlate Method. You can download it for free here: https://mail.fromthestartnutrition.com/get-secret-to-end-mealtime-battles-6930

References

"Postpartum Nutrition." Cleveland Clinic, my.clevelandclinic.org/health/articles/21508-postpartum-nutrition. Accessed 29 Dec 2023.

"How to Use The Plate Method for Meal Planning." Nutrition with Megan, https://www.fromthestartnutrition.com. Accessed 29 Dec 2023.

https://www.healthychildren.org/English/ages-stages/baby/feeding-nutrition/Pages/how-often-and-how-much-should-your-baby-eat.aspx. Accessed 29 Dec 2023.

"How Often and How Much Should Your Baby Eat?" Healthy Children, American Academy of Pediatrics, www.healthychildren.org/English/ages-stages/baby/feeding-nutrition/Pages/how-often-and-how-much-should-your-baby-eat.aspx. Accessed 29 Dec 2023.

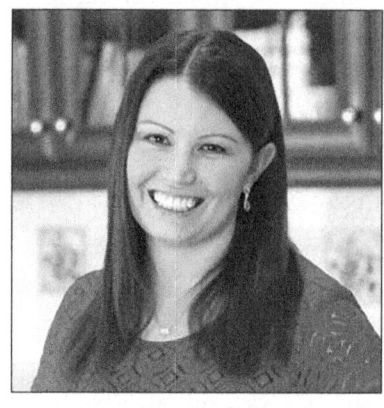

Beth Conlon, PhD, RDN, is a Pediatric and Family Dietitian with over 14 years of experience as a Registered Dietitian Nutritionist combined with a PhD in Clinical Investigation plus personal experiences as a mom of four. She provides clients with nutrition therapy and counseling backed by the latest science-based research. Beth is particularly passionate about family-based nutrition interventions for children and teens and has produced over 12 peer-reviewed academic publications in this area. In addition, she completed Postdoctoral training in the Medical Nutrition Industry at Nestle Health Science and has served as a University assistant and adjunct professor for over five years.

Beth is passionate about helping children and families grow and thrive through good nutrition. She founded From the Start Nutrition, LLC, in 2020 to pursue her mission of empowering families everywhere to make informed food choices that promote health and wellbeing, while also fostering a positive and lifelong relationship with food, body, and self.

In her free time, you'll find Beth playing with her kids, attending a Barre class or doing a home YouTube exercise video, walking her Australian Shepherd, and enjoying black coffee and chocolates.

If you would like additional support for your postpartum nutrition journey, whether for yourself, your baby, or both, get in touch with Beth today to schedule a free consultation at www.fromthestartnutrition.com.

Connect with Beth:

Website: https://www.fromthestartnutrition.com

LinkedIn: https://www.linkedin.com/in/bethconlon

Facebook: https://www.Facebook.com/fromthestartnutrition

Instagram: https://www.Instagram.com/fromthestartnutrition

Twitter: https://www.Twitter.com/fromthestartrdn

YouTube: https://www.youtube.com/@fromthestartnutrition

CHAPTER 15

Planning Ahead with Your Estate Planning

CREATING A PLAN FOR YOUR FAMILY

Valerie E. Anias, Esq., Founder of A Team Family Law, LLC

It's a whirlwind. You find out you're pregnant, compare your growing fetus to various fruits and vegetables, finally figure out what you can eat until the smell knocks it off the "safe" list, and plan for the birth (the actual birth never goes as planned).

Then there's the hospital stay with very little sleep and getting to know this new human. I remember when the nurses took us back to the maternity room. There we were with our child, and all I can remember thinking is:

Now what?

They are just going to leave them here?

What do we do now?

It was not the lack of maternal instinct. I felt comfortable with my child and my ability to take care of them. I felt the incredible and indescribable love in those moments. It was more this feeling of something greater. I knew that I now had this immense amount of responsibility, and frankly, I did not know what to do with that.

Then, the intrusive thoughts:

What happens if I'm not here?

What happens if my partner isn't here?

What happens if…

Those are the worst. The thoughts of something horrible happening. The most horrible thought of your baby being alone:

What happens to them?

Foster care?

What about providing for them?

Who will take on that responsibility?

I felt a bit silly if I'm being honest. I was a lawyer. I knew, at the very least, exactly what I needed to do to protect my child and future children. And, even as a lawyer, I felt the weight of those thoughts. Even as a lawyer, I felt confused, overwhelmed, and frozen. It can make you lose sleep. It made me lose sleep.

My goal is to help you avoid sleepless nights in at least one aspect. Between my own experience and understanding and my profession, I can help you answer those questions. I can help you avoid the alternative: ignoring the problem.

At some point, it seems that many parents learn to ignore this intrusive voice and push through. Maybe it's the lack of sleep, the ever-changing sleep schedule and recommendations, this swaddle versus that swaddle. All the other thoughts take priority in their brain and mute the intrusive voice. Not every problem has an immediate solution. Not every intrusive thought has an answer. But what if there was a way to resolve the intrusive voices rather than silence them?

There have been several occasions where I have had new parents on their consultation call absolutely petrified about what would happen with their kids if they and their co-parent were to suddenly die. Most often their concerns happen to surround some sort of tragic event.

"We're going on a trip. What happens if the plane crashes while we're *both* on it?!"

"I have a work trip; my co-parent drives to and from the office; what if we both don't make it home to our child?!"

There is no Magic 8 Ball™ that is going to tell all parents when and how they will die and what will happen to their kids. The good news is that you can create your own "Magic 8 Ball™," so to speak. You may not know how or when you'll pass, but you can dictate your wishes and make them known. You can plan for your family. You can create a plan for your children.

I founded A Team Family Law, LLC because I wanted to have a family-focused, family-centered law firm. Estate Planning is an area of law that I believe belongs under the Family Law umbrella. By planning ahead with your Estate Plan, you are, in fact, planning for your family. When your Estate Plan is in use, you're no longer able to make decisions. This does not necessarily mean you're deceased. It could mean you're cognitively impaired or otherwise unable to make decisions. The importance is that *you* created the Estate Plan while you were able so that when you're unable, your family can continue to do as you wished. Those intrusive questions? Answered. The "What if…" "How will I…" "Who will my children…" Answered.

So, how do you create your own "Magic 8 Ball™?" By creating your own Estate Plan. The amount of relief you feel once you have your bases covered is felt by everyone. When my clients come in and do their final signing of these documents, there is almost always an audible sigh of relief.

Before we dive into the various factors that make Estate Planning particularly relevant for parents, we need to clarify, define, and explain the ambiguity of an "Estate Plan."

THE BASICS

Estate Planning refers to the process of ensuring that an individual's wishes are carried out. An individual's "wishes" can mean their property, real estate, how they want to be buried, what happens to that grandfather clock that has been passed down from generation to generation, who gets great-grandma's jewelry, what song is played at their funeral, and whether their organs will be donated. Of relevance and importance to parents, it also includes designations for guardians of their minor children and an avenue to financially plan for their children.

When individuals refer to their Estate Plan, it could include a variety of different components. Key components could include:

Last Will & Testament: This is the legal document that outlines how an individual's assets will be distributed upon their death. It also includes guardianship designation for minor children and any other specific wishes parents may have. This document only becomes effective upon an individual's death.

Trusts: These arrangements allow a third party, referred to as a trustee, to hold and manage assets on behalf of those designated to be a recipient of that benefit, referred to as beneficiaries. Trusts can avoid probate, provide for minor children, or manage assets for individuals with special needs.

Power of Attorney: This is a legal document that grants someone the authority to make medical or financial decisions on behalf of an individual in the event they become unable to do so.

Many individuals believe that only the wealthy need an Estate Plan. False. Having a pulse makes you a great candidate for creating your Estate Plan. Being of a sound mind makes you a great candidate for creating your Estate Plan. There's no financial threshold to meet. There is just you, an individual who has wishes. Now, an individual who has a child and wants to protect their family.

ESTATE PLANNING WITH MINOR CHILDREN

Estate Planning is especially crucial for people with minor children. Remember those intrusive thoughts? Estate Planning helps ensure the well-being and financial security of your children. This is your Magic 8 Ball™. Estate Planning with your children in mind will help alleviate the "what ifs" by providing the answers.

What can you answer with Estate Planning when you have minor children? The Big Three:

1. **WHO** will care for my children?
2. **HOW** will they be provided for?
3. **WHEN** should I start planning?

WHO: THE GUARDIANSHIP DESIGNATION

Estate Planning allows parents to designate a legal guardian for their minor children in the event that both parents pass away. This ensures that the children will be cared for by individuals chosen by you rather than leaving the decision to the Court

By designating a legal guardian for your minor children in your Estate Plan, you have the opportunity to express your wishes regarding who you believe is the most suitable person or persons to care for your children. While you and your co-parent may not be here to raise your children, this designation gives you and your co-parent the control to make a decision that is in accordance with your values and beliefs.

Clear guardianship instructions can help prevent potential family disputes over who should have custody of the children. Your children have already suffered a tremendous loss. The idea of legal battles between various family members in disagreement about who will care for your children is only added stress for the children.

Without a designated guardian, the Court will have to determine who will care for your children in the event of your passing. That process can be time-consuming and emotionally challenging, especially if there are family disputes. Designating a guardian in advance with your Estate Plan allows you to avoid Court intervention and ensures a smoother transition for your children. It also allows those whom you've appointed time to ask questions, ensure they understand the process in the event of a tragedy, and, most importantly, to be made aware of your wishes or where they can find your Estate Plan.

Estate Planning allows you to consider various factors when selecting a person or persons to be guardian(s) for your minor children. You can consider the potential guardian(s) values, parenting style, religious and/or moral beliefs, family life, number of kids, and their physical location. This ensures your children will be raised in an environment that aligns with your preferences.

The death of a parent is a traumatizing and challenging time for children. Knowing who will care for them in the event of this situation provides children with a sense of stability. It helps minimize the disruption and emotional trauma that may result from sudden changes in their living arrangements. Additionally, it provides clear instructions to your family and mitigates potential disputes.

HOW: FINANCIAL SUPPORT AND DISTRIBUTION

Creating your Estate Plan offers a comprehensive approach to managing the financial aspects of your estate, particularly when there are minor children involved.

Estate Planning allows you, the parents, to determine how your assets will be distributed among your children. Through Estate Planning tools like wills and trusts, you can specify terms under which your children will inherit their assets, which will ensure that the distribution aligns with your financial goals and values.

Some parents decide to create a trust for the benefit of their children. Trusts can be structured to hold and manage assets on behalf of your children until they reach a certain age or achieve a specific milestone. This helps protect and grow the assets for the benefit of the children, especially if parents pass when they're very young. Some trusts are specifically created for certain situations.

Estate Planning provides parents an opportunity to set aside funds earmarked for specific occasions such as education. This may involve creating educational trusts or utilizing tax-advantaged accounts, such as 529 plans, to ensure there are resources available for your children's academic expenses. Some trusts are created for children who have special needs. Special provisions can be made to ensure that the child's unique financial needs are met without jeopardizing their ability to remain eligible or become eligible for government benefits.

Life insurance is often a crucial component of your Estate Plan. Having a life insurance plan for yourself and your co-parent can provide a financial safety net for the surviving family members. Because life insurance proceeds pay out quickly, these funds can be used to cover immediate expenses such as mortgage payments, education costs, or other immediate expenses necessary to mitigate the instability in your children's lives.

By strategically planning the distribution of assets, utilizing tools, and incorporating life insurance, you can provide a solid foundation for your children's financial future well-being. The fear of how your children will be provided for by those you have selected to care for them is a burden you do not have to carry.

WHEN: CREATING YOUR ESTATE PLAN

Many individuals, including parents, believe creating your Estate Plan should happen after some sort of financial threshold is met. This is untrue. All individuals should create their Estate Plan as soon as possible. Parents who do not have an Estate Plan prior to having children should consider Estate Planning as soon as they have minor children. Timing is essential as unexpected events can happen. Having a comprehensive Estate Plan in place provides a safety net for the well-being of both the parents and their children. Below are some key milestones and considerations parents may consider.

Ideally, Estate Planning should begin with the birth of your first child. This is the point at which you should start thinking about the future financial and legal aspects of your family. While it may seem early, having a plan in place offers peace of mind and quiets those "what if" questions. Having additional children does not necessarily require making amendments to any Estate Plan unless there are specific requests or unique considerations you may wish to include as it relates to those specific children.

As discussed above, upon the birth of your child(ren), you may designate legal guardians for them. In the event of death, the nominated guardians will be able to take immediate action to ensure the well-being of your children. This decision is critical, and you should have a clear understanding of who you would want to care for your children if both parents were unable to do so.

While at the birth of your first child, you may not have accumulated much in the way of assets, this may not ring true five or ten years later. As you accumulate assets, whether through homeownership, investments, or other means, the complexity of your financial situation increases. Estate Planning allows you to outline how these assets should be distributed, ensuring that your children are provided for in the best possible way.

The birth of your first child or the expansion of your family is an opportune time for you to begin the Estate Planning process. Starting early and regularly updating the plan, if needed, ensures that it remains relevant and effective in addressing the ever-evolving needs of your family. It is never too early to start planning for the future and providing security for your family.

NOW WHAT?

You know a bit more about Estate Planning. You know a bit more about why it is important to have a plan when you have minor children. Now what?

1. Talk with your co-parent about individuals who embody the values and principles that you would want for your children.
2. Talk with your co-parent about specific items that may be of importance (ex., a specific piece of jewelry, a piece of furniture, etc.).
3. Talk with your co-parent about financial matters you find important (ex., an education fund, what age is appropriate for children to receive any kind of cash or distribution, etc.).

Once you have these considerations written down, consider other matters you may deem important. For example, obtaining a life insurance policy for immediate funds, how you intend to notify individuals of their specific roles, and your timeline for ensuring these considerations are encapsulated in your Estate Plan. After you've had the conversation and taken these notes, reach out to an Estate Planning attorney. An attorney will ensure your wishes are represented in your Estate Plan. An attorney will ensure that any additional considerations are brought to your attention. An attorney will ensure compliance with the law so your wishes can come to fruition.

It's important to know that creating your Estate Plan now doesn't mean you cannot change it later. Amending your Estate Plan is often necessary to ensure that the documents remain aligned with your family's evolving circumstances and preferences. Life is dynamic, marked by changes in relationships, financial status, and personal priorities. Once you have created your Estate Plan, individuals should periodically review their plan and consider any amendments. Whether the amendments are prompted by a significant life event or simply a desire to redefine your wishes, amending your Estate Plan offers flexibility to reflect your wishes. Regularly revisiting and amending your Estate Plan demonstrates a commitment to maintaining a comprehensive and up-to-date strategy that best serves you and your family.

The process of Estate Planning for parents with children is a crucial and multifaceted endeavor that goes beyond the mere distribution of assets. It can be overwhelming, challenging, and even frightening. However, it can also be empowering, relieving, and create a sense of security. From crafting a comprehensive will to establishing trusts and designating guardians, the complexities of Estate Planning demand thoughtful attention. By addressing potential challenges and fostering open communication within your family, you can create a legacy that not only preserves your hard-earned assets but also provides a stable foundation for your children's future. Ultimately, this chapter underscores the importance of proactive planning, ensuring that an already difficult transition is made as seamless as possible. Most importantly, creating an Estate Plan serves as a testament to your enduring commitment to your family. After all, you are creating an Estate Plan for your family.

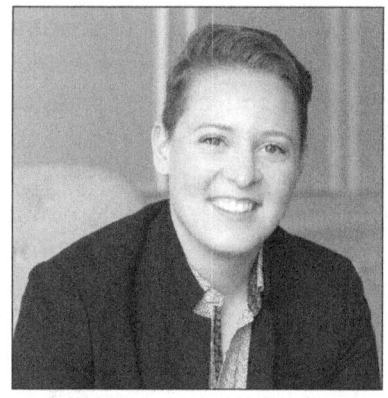

Valerie E. Anias, Esq., is the founder of A Team Family Law, LLC, where she focuses her practice on family-related matters such as divorce, custody, adoption, and Estate Planning. Val brings compassion, understanding, and thoroughness to the table when taking on a case. She is passionate about assisting underrepresented individuals and advocates for her clients irrespective of their gender, race, sexual orientation, family status, etc. Whether the issue involves a child custody dispute, divorce, adoption, or creating your Estate Plan, Val's approach provides her clients with top-notch legal representation and ensures that her clients' rights and voices are represented passionately and efficiently.

Val is originally from New York (and will always remain a Yankee fan) and moved to Maryland in 2012 for law school at the University of Baltimore School of Law. When not practicing law, you will find Val spending time with her family, enjoying a cup of coffee, taking a hike, or finding some other unique gem to explore with her wife and kids. Val lives in Anne Arundel County with her wife, kids, and two dogs.

To reach out to Val and learn more about A Team Family Law, LLC:

Website: https://ateamfamilylaw.com/

Facebook: https://www.facebook.com/ateamfamilylaw

Instagram: https://www.instagram.com/ateamfamilylaw/

LinkedIn: https://www.linkedin.com/in/valerie-e-anias-esq-bb162a32/

CHAPTER 16

Sweeping Away Chaos

SIMPLE STEPS TO KEEP YOUR SPACE CLEAN AND ORGANIZED

Kaitlyn Martin and Shelly Schoff,
Co-Owners of Crabtown Cleaning

OUR STORY

As a mother-daughter team working together and navigating different parenting stages, we created this chapter based on our unique blend of wisdom and insight from very distinct parenting perspectives. Our shared passion for creating chaos-free and organized home environments unites our vision and allows us to share practical tips and strategies we've adopted in our own homes. These strategies help us find balance in the beautiful chaos that exists at every stage of motherhood. We hope you apply these suggestions to find peace and harmony in your home.

From Kaitlyn's perspective - as a new mom of two under two, I found myself lost in the chaos of diapers, bottles, and sleepless nights. While the joy of welcoming my second son was evident, the stress and anxiety around my chaotic home was overwhelming. I'm sure many moms can relate.

When my first son was born, I felt like I had no responsibility. I reminded myself that I was a first-time mom and needed to give myself some grace. I spent most of my days holding my new baby boy. We spent lots of time cuddling on the couch and let the laundry and clutter in the house pile up without a second thought.

Soon after my son turned one, we found out we were pregnant with our second child. We knew our small rancher was not going to cut it for a family of four. We spent hours back and forth about what the right thing to do was. We even looked at moving, but we love our home. Of course, my husband didn't find an issue with living in a tiny home. Boy, was he wrong!

Ultimately, we made the decision to build an addition. It truly was the best decision we could have made for our growing family. Along with this addition came new space and organization - which was awesome. We spent the weeks before the birth of our second son sorting through everything. We reorganized our entire home and implemented many of the strategies mentioned in our chapter.

Most days, we stick to it. But we aren't perfect, and sometimes we fall short. Our kids are way too young to include them in the cleaning, so for now, it's just my husband and me. It's not hard to stay motivated because we know it's crucial, and when we keep up, we don't find piles building up on the dining room table, which seems to be our catchall. And we don't find ourselves running out of underwear anymore.

Yes, it is 15 minutes I could spend relaxing, scrolling through social media, sleeping, or just sitting and talking to my husband. But instead, we choose tranquility in our home. Those 15 minutes have made such a difference in the daily, weekly, monthly, and bi-annual chores. Waking up in the morning and not having to clean up before making breakfast for the babies is so worth the 15-minute sacrifice.

From Shelly's perspective - As a veteran mom with adult children, I've experienced many seasons of motherhood. The newborn phase was always exceptionally challenging, and as a mom who worked outside the home full-time, it was especially important to keep up with household chores on a regular basis. Time was always at a premium, and we couldn't afford to let things get behind.

My nightly reset routine is my favorite strategy, and it was inspired by my mom, whom the grandkids call Mimi. She was the hardest-working and most caring person I have ever known, and she absolutely loved having her home neat and orderly. As a working mom of three and Mimi to three grandkids, she had a lot on her plate. I still remember her being up late at night when we were kids. Way past everyone else because she was working to get all the dishes done, make sure we all had clean laundry for the next day, and pull together everything we needed to get out of the house on time in the morning. As a kid, it never dawned on me that she probably could have used our help. She made it seem effortless, even though now, as an adult, I know she was probably exhausted. But she never complained and rarely asked for help. My memories of her working her nightly routine night after night inspire me to keep going even when I'm tired and feel like skipping out to relax in front of my favorite television show. Mimi was a breast cancer survivor and passed away in 2016 after a long battle with heart disease. She was the inspiration for our business start-up and the reason we are so passionate about our dedication to providing free cleaning services to patients battling cancer. She was an amazing, strong woman, a fantastic mom and role model, and I miss her terribly. I am so thankful she instilled in me the value of keeping my home neat and organized.

Many of the systems we implemented over the years have been carried forward into our daughter's home as well. By sharing these tips and strategies with you we hope you are able to easily maintain your home and spend less time and mental energy worrying about your housework and more time enjoying your family and doing the things you love.

THE TOOL

Congratulations on your new arrival! As you start the incredible journey of motherhood, creating a clutter-free and organized home can make all the difference in maintaining your sanity so you can truly enjoy the precious moments with your little ones. In this chapter, we'll explore practical and purposeful ways to transform your home into a peaceful, tranquil space in seven simple steps.

STEP 1: THE POWER OF PURPOSEFUL SPACES

The first step in calming the clutter is recognizing the magic that purposeful spaces can bring to your home. Imagine living in a home where every item has a designated spot. Can you see it? Suddenly, the chaos is replaced by peace and harmony. The truth is, it's easier than you may think to attain this goal, and it's not just about tidying up; it's about assigning meaning and purpose to every nook and cranny of your home.

Making a Mindset Shift

Before you can even get started, you'll need to shift your mindset. Stop looking at decluttering as an overwhelming task and start seeing it as an opportunity to create personal space in your home that nurtures both you and your growing family. Embrace the idea that every item in your home serves a purpose and deserves a home of its own.

Identify Your Problem Areas

Take a few moments and walk through your home with a notepad. Stop in each problem area and consider what you see in that area that causes you stress or anxiety. Take notes and try to identify what tends to get clogged or bottlenecked with clutter. These areas might include your entranceway, a kitchen table or island, a pantry, or a playroom. Create a list of all the cluttered areas you feel contribute to the chaos in your home.

Define Zones

Once you have identified the problem areas, take some time to think about how you can define specific zones to create a designated space to contain and control items causing the clutter. If your entranceway is full of backpacks, mail, and keys, think about where you can create a drop zone for these items. Visualize what that space might look like. Do you need hooks on the wall for backpacks and keys? Do you need a crate or a bench to house everyone's shoes? A bin to hold the incoming mail? Make a list of the items you need to create an orderly space with a designated spot for every item.

Once you have your list, work on finding and installing these items. In our home, the solution for our entranceway was a hall tree we ordered from Amazon for about $90. It has hooks across the top and a few shelves across the bottom. It works perfectly to keep our families' clutter contained—no need to create elaborate or expensive solutions. Your items can be as simple as a few command strips for the hooks and a recycled box for the mail, but once you gain confidence in finding solutions for one zone, the ideas will flow more easily for each new zone you create.

Remember, you don't have to do everything all at once. Create one or two functional zones every month, and before you know it, you'll work your way through your entire list of problem areas. Creating purposeful spaces for every item in your home will lay the foundation for a clutter-free sanctuary that brings you peace and joy.

STEP 2: THE FREEDOM OF LETTING GO

Now that we've embraced the idea of creating purposeful spaces, let's talk about the elephant in the room—too much stuff! It's tough to create a designated space for every item if your home is jammed full of personal belongings. One of the greatest rules we've adopted in our home is to look critically at our space periodically to identify any items that do not have a home and make the decision to toss them.

The Three Box Technique

When creating new zones in your home, be sure to find space for a Declutter Zone. This area should include three boxes: one memory box for items to keep, one box for donations, and one box for things to toss. As you work through each room of your home, be vigilant in your decision-making. If an item doesn't have a home or a purpose, place it in one of these three boxes. Implementing this practice not only declutters your home but also pays it forward to others who may have a use for the items that no longer serve you.

Embrace Your Emotions

You may find yourself struggling with your emotions as you consider letting go of items that are sentimental or emotionally tied to your little ones. It's okay to feel that connection but remember many of these items have served their purpose for your family and can still be enjoyed by others. For items that are especially important, keep them in your memories box. But for other items, consider taking a photo as a keepsake and then let them go so they can bring joy to others.

Streamline Your Digital Space

Don't forget to address your digital clutter too! Your physical space is not the only area that'll better serve you without the clutter. We all spend so much time on our devices these days. It's worth investing some time to clean up your digital space. Searching for documents, apps, or photos can be extremely frustrating when your digital files are disorganized. Grab a coffee and spend a quiet morning clearing out your emails, sorting through your photos, and organizing your documents. Be sure to delete what is no longer needed and organize everything else into files and folders.

Reminder! Don't forget to take time to appreciate the progress you've made. Celebrate each victory, no matter how small. These small changes will add up over time. Remember, decluttering is a journey, not a sprint.

STEP 3: DELETE THE DUPLICATES

As a new mom, you can quickly become inundated with baby gear. Don't let the overwhelm of these items create new clutter in your life. If your drawers and closets are bursting at the seams, you probably have more baby gear than you actually need.

Assess Your Inventory

Start by sorting everything into categories so you can quickly tell if you have more than you need. Onesies are great, but if you have fifteen sizes 0-3 months, consider keeping just what you can use and donate the rest. Start by sorting like items into categories so you can easily identify duplicates. Any duplicate items should be donated to a local charity or a family in need.

Organize What You Keep

Once you remove duplicates, sort the remaining items strategically. Keep similar items grouped together. Storing like items together will make it easier to recognize when duplicates show up in the future and will allow you to quickly identify and remove them.

Learn to Say No

As a new mom, you'll likely have an abundance of offers from well-meaning family and friends wanting to share hand-me-downs from their children. While support from your community is wonderful and appreciated, if the items offered are duplicates of things you already have, it's okay to graciously decline. Let them know you sincerely appreciate their offer but believe it would be best to pass the items along to someone with a greater need.

A great way to find families in need of the items you have to offer is to join a local Facebook group. When our oldest child started to outgrow his newborn clothes, we were able to find a local "Buy Nothing, Sell Nothing" group in our community. To find these groups in your area, just jump on Facebook and search Buy Nothing Sell Nothing with the name of your local town or community included in the search. This has been an amazing resource and a wonderful way to meet and connect with other local families.

STEP 4: MAINTAINING THE BALANCE

Now that we've purged duplicates, tossed everything that didn't have a home, created zones, and established a designated space for every item, how do we keep it this way? The answer—by carefully managing and intentionally selecting new items we bring into our home.

Adopt a One-In One-Out Rule

You've worked hard to make sure everything has a designated space. Your home looks great, and you want to keep it that way. The best way to keep clutter from building back up is to remove one similar item for every new item you bring into your home. New gloves for Christmas? Toss last year's gloves. New brown boots? Donate the old pair. If you consistently apply this rule for every new item that enters your home, it will be easy to maintain the progress you've made.

The Magic of Toy Rotation

Let's face it: kids get bored easily. That's why they have tons of toys in the first place. Do they play with all of them every day? No way! Here's a simple trick to keep your toy room under control. Only give your kids access to half of their toys. Buy a huge storage tub, load it up with half the toys lying around, and put them in storage for a month. Suddenly, it's easy to put away all the toys because now there is space for everything. Your kids will never even notice anything is missing. Thirty days from now, pull out the bin, swap the toys, and the kids will think it's

Christmas. They'll be excited to play with something new, and you'll have an easier job cleaning up the playroom.

Learning to Go With The Flow

As with anything in life, there will be seasons when things are easier to maintain and seasons when things are more difficult. A new puppy or a lengthy illness may throw off even the best-laid plans. If you are in a season of difficult times, be kind to yourself and give yourself some grace. If you fall behind in keeping up with your tasks, know you can start back anytime. By laying this foundation, it will be easy to pick up where you left off and get back on track.

STEP 5: YOUR NIGHTLY RESET

As we dive deeper into living in the bliss of a clutter-free home, we invite you to embrace a new game-changing habit of ending each day with a nightly reset routine. Imagine waking up in the morning to a peaceful and tranquil home that was restored to order before bedtime the night before.

15-Minute Power Play

Before you head off to bed, set an alarm and complete as many targeted tasks as possible in this time frame. Throw in a load of laundry, load dishes in the dishwasher, pack tomorrow's lunches, and lay out your clothes for tomorrow. Better yet, involve the whole family. With a family of four, you'll squeeze an hour of chores into a 15-minute timespan. Making this a daily habit you follow consistently will change your life for the better.

Clearing the Kitchen

The kitchen is the heart of every home, so make sure your nightly routine includes a quick tidy in this area. Clear countertops, wipe surfaces, and load the dishes into the dishwasher. This will not take long, and starting your day with a clutter-free kitchen will set the tone for the next day.

Peaceful Sleep Environment

Before you jump into bed, look around and make sure what you will see when you wake up is visually pleasing. Hang up any clothes lying around, fold blankets not being used, throw away trash, and put away your technology. Eliminating anything that might cause stress or anxiety as you wake up lays the groundwork for a great start to the day.

STEP 6: FOLLOW YOUR HOT MOM'S CLEAN ROUTINE GUIDE TO CLUTTER CONTROL

It's easy to get lost in the overwhelm of where to start, so we've created our Clean Routine Guide to help you on your journey to gaining control over the clutter in your home. The guide provides a physical tool that gives a quick visual of the tasks you've already completed and the remaining tasks. The tool is broken down into five sections: Daily, Weekly, Biweekly, Monthly, and Biannual tasks. You'll be able to customize your tasks into a simple schedule that works best for you.

The Power of Consistency

Consistency is the best way to succeed in keeping your home clean and clutter-free. Our guide provides checks and balances that will help you stay focused.

Cleaning Tasks

Creating your customized recurring cleaning routine will help you spread your cleaning tasks into small, manageable tasks, motivating you to keep working through the list to achieve your goals.

Decluttering Tasks

Keeping up with your decluttering tasks on an ongoing basis ensures they will never become an overwhelming chore again.

STEP 7: MOVING FORWARD WITH A QUARTERLY ROUTINE

The final step of our clutter-busting journey is to ensure we are ready to change and adapt to new challenges. To ensure we recognize when change is necessary, we'll need to monitor and review our routine at least once every quarter.

Set Aside Time to Reflect

Once each quarter, schedule some quiet time to reflect on your progress. Have you finished creating all the zones you wanted to create? Take another walk through your home. This time, think about how each new zone is functioning. Is it serving its purpose? Is it easy to clean? Are there changes or adjustments needed? Plan to implement changes in any zone that is not working well.

Be Open to Change

Motherhood is fluid, and things will change. Kids will grow, and routines will change. Don't let this catch you off guard or fool you into thinking your efforts are not paying off. Change is natural. Embrace the change and incorporate new strategies. When your kids start playing sports, you may need to create a new drop zone for sports equipment. Use the principles learned here to create a new solution to manage and contain the sports equipment. Eventually, creating space for every new challenge will become second nature.

Build A Reward System

A clean and clutter-free home is an amazing reward, but keeping up with these tasks may require additional motivation. Brainstorm to find a reward system to help you stay the course. Encourage your spouse to get on board by scheduling a date night as a reward for completing your Nightly Reset Routine together for thirty days.

Celebrate your progress! As we wrap up our seven Simple Steps to Keep Your Space Clean and Organized, we hope you will stop and recognize the progress you've made. You've worked hard and deserve to take a moment to reflect on your accomplishments. Thank you for coming along with us on this journey! May your home be filled with love, laughter, joy, and all the delightful things that motherhood has to offer.

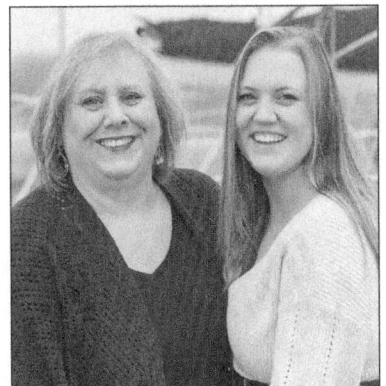

Kaitlyn Martin, Co-Owner, with a B.S. in Psychology and a minor in Elementary Education from Palm Beach Atlantic University. Kaitlyn transitioned from the classroom to join the family business and work alongside her mother. Her passion for creating clean and organized spaces fuels Crabtown's commitment to creating *Clean Happy Spaces*.

Shelly Schoff, Co-Owner, brings over three decades of expertise from the financial services industry to Crabtown Cleaning. With precise attention to detail and strong organizational skills, she has designed operational procedures and customer service standards that exemplify excellence in the residential cleaning industry.

Together, Kaitlyn and Shelly are on a mission to transform not only the physical space of Annapolis homes but also to have a positive impact on the families they serve! Their insights and practical advice in this chapter aim to empower new moms in navigating the joys and demands of motherhood.

A common passion shared by both Kaitlyn and Shelly is giving back to their community by donating time to clean homes for cancer patients through their partnership with Cleaning For A Reason. To learn more about this organization and find out how you can support their efforts, please follow the link below.

Connect with Kaitlyn and Shelly:

Website: https://www.crabtowncleaning.com
Facebook: https://www.Facebook.com/crabtowncleaning
Instagram: https://www.Instagram.com/crabtowncleaning
Learn More About Cleaning For A Reason: https://cleaningforareason.org
Visit our website at
https://www.crabtowncleaning.com/cleanroutineguide to download your free copy of our Clean Routine Guide for Clutter Control

CHAPTER 17

Replenishing Wholeness

RESTORING THE MIND, BODY, AND SOUL CONNECTION AFTER CHILDBIRTH

Dr. Irum Tahir

There I was, staring at the bright lights of the emergency room ceiling at 2 a.m., asking myself, *How did **I** get **here**?* The truth was, I wasn't quite sure. Before I was dropped off at the ER, I had trouble swallowing and breathing and felt all my muscles weaken; I couldn't even walk up the short flight of stairs at home without straining and not being able to breathe.

I called my dad, who is a physician, and asked him what I should do, and he said, "Go straight to the ER." While at the ER, they couldn't figure out where my symptoms were coming from and sent me home; I was terrified. From that moment, I had every blood test, imaging, and testing possible in order to find out what was wrong and why I felt the way I did. I was once a vibrant and very active doctor, seeing multiple patients a day. At this point, I could only see about five patients a day and was too exhausted to perform chiropractic adjustments. I slept or laid down between visits.

I racked my brain, thinking about what could possibly be going on with my body, all the while scared of what "it" could be. The only thing I could think of was that I was cleaning up a polluted lake in our area for Earth Day and was bit by a tiny black worm, and after that, my symptoms began. Before the bite, I had been tired and exhausted for some time, but that bite took my body over the edge, and I landed in the ER.

I'm forever grateful to have found a great associate doctor to see my patients and continue to grow the practice I built while I focused on healing myself.

What was wrong? After all the testing and going to medical specialists and experts locally and nationally with no answers, I was overwhelmed and frustrated. Finally, I decided that if there was a chance of recovery, I'd have to do it on my own and, "Doctor, first, heal thyself."

I set my healing in motion beginning with what I knew—chiropractic care three times a week to reset my nervous system and release tension. I researched and learned everything I could about anti-inflammatory and detox protocols to naturally detoxify my body, and I figured out I had adrenal fatigue, which I'd been pushing through for quite some time as I built my business. I used healing modalities such as acupuncture, eating fresh, organic foods, and physical therapy. I found ways to heal and nurture myself—something I veered so far from—and my body responded beautifully! I'm so grateful to say that with the right attention, direction, and focus—and with God's Grace—my body healed naturally. It took a good year and a half, but I began to feel better than I thought possible. Through this experience, I was able to reconnect my mind, body, and soul and now have helped tens of thousands of women in all stages of life do the same.

THE TOOL

MOTHERHOOD

We often disconnect from our own mind, body, and soul when our motherhood journey begins. It's that maternal connection that binds us to this beautiful creation in our lives, and suddenly, everything else just seems not that important compared to what is right in front of us.

I've had the immense privilege of being a part of the healthcare of tens of thousands of moms and completing 100,000+ visits as a Chiropractor all over the world, from working with women who have survived war in Syria and living in refugee camps in Jordan, to mothers in India, Madagascar, Syracuse, New York and Annapolis, Maryland. And I've seen a recurring pattern of motherhood—moms, especially new moms, put themselves *last*.

As necessary as it may seem in the moment (or it seems that it's just what's required at the time), a negative cycle can be created, where a deep lack of self-care and unmet physical, mental, and emotional needs added to changes and shifts in the body can create an environment of burnout and even resentment. What can exacerbate issues further is there are physical, mental, and emotional challenges that have not been resolved or the mom was unaware of even before getting pregnant. As I tell my patients, pregnancy can magnify underlying conditions and issues, and it can only make it all more challenging if not taken care of early on. In this chapter, I'll help you restore that mind, body, and soul connection and ultimately reconnect to yourself and who you really are, no matter what stage of motherhood you're in.

Let's start with the body because everything begins with how you feel in the home that you're living in, which is your physical being.

Pregnancy creates a change in the biomechanics of the spine and pelvis. As pregnancy progresses and the baby grows, an anterior pelvic tilt occurs, creating a hyperlordosis in the lumbar spine and an increased kyphosis in the thoracic spine with a possible forward head carriage. This posture can worsen through the pregnancy and into the postpartum with nursing or childcare. These issues may have started up during the pregnancy itself and were never addressed or minimized.

Since many pregnant women are often told that the pain or discomfort they may be experiencing is a natural part of pregnancy and there aren't many solutions, many of the complaints pregnant moms actually have might never have been addressed and will then follow them through the pregnancy, labor, and delivery, and possibly into the postpartum period. Complaints may get worse with each subsequent pregnancy, labor, delivery, and postpartum period.

There are several physical complaints you could imagine relate to an anterior pelvic tilt and the changes in the lumbopelvic biomechanics, such as low back pain, sciatica, sacroiliac joint dysfunction, pubic symphysis pain, and round ligament pain, but the change in biomechanics of the body, especially the pelvis, can also result in a change or increase in neck pain, headaches, and thoracic pain.

Since the pelvis is the foundation of the body and all the vertebrae of the body sit on top of it, pelvic or SI joint dysfunction can cause a cascade effect through the entire body, and the spine attempts to correct itself due to the imbalance and stress of an unleveled or tilted foundation.

My specialization is to address the low back and pelvis by checking nine structures to ascertain exactly where an issue is coming from, and heal it with Chiropractic care. My belief is that by getting to the root of the issue and addressing it from the core, the body can finally heal and feel well.

In practice, I see these issues so often, and the postpartum mom may be in chronic pain. By the time she enters my office, she has tried all sorts of therapies, some of which have helped, some have gotten her to a plateau, others keep the pain away for a longer period of time, and others a shorter window of time. I'd urge anyone who is in pain or has discomfort to address the issue sooner rather than later.

ACHIEVING YOUR PHYSICAL HEALTH GOALS

The first thing you need to do is sit in a quiet place and scan your body. Ask yourself, where are you holding pain, tenderness, or tension? How long have you been holding this? When was the first time you felt this pain or discomfort? How is this impacting your activities of daily living? What is your stress level? How is it impacting you, your body, or your loved ones? What are you not able to do that you would like to do? Is there more than one complaint?

If there are many complaints, go through the process again and prioritize what is the worst (affecting you more or the issue has been there longer) to the least. I've found it actually helps to write it down in order of priority. Once we have this information, we want to be able to determine who can help you in addition to your medical team. There are so many resources right in this book, from postpartum Chiropractors, physical therapists, personal trainers, dietitians, and more.

We all know eating well is important. In the postpartum phase, there may be a depletion of nutrients; after all, your body is creating another little body. Even if you've gotten the correct nutrients and supplementation during pregnancy, your body can still be depleted in many ways. Shifting your attention to consuming whole organic foods, good levels of protein, and plenty of fresh water will do wonders for the body.

My patients have done well by adding organic bone broths to their daily regimen as well as nourishing soups and stews often able to be made ahead of time. Greatly reducing or eliminating sugar and alcohol and minimizing caffeine can also be very replenishing during the postpartum phase.

I've found in working with the postpartum mom that magnesium glycinate, omega-3 fatty acids, and Vitamin D can make a shift for the postpartum body. Either taking these as supplements or adding magnesium-rich foods such as spinach, omega-3-rich foods such as high-quality wild-caught fish, or sardines and nuts can be very helpful! Please make sure to check with your healthcare provider before beginning any new supplements to ensure they are appropriate for your specific needs.

REPLENISHING YOUR SOUL

Stress has been linked to almost every chronic disease. We're all told to manage our stress better, but if we're in a chronic cycle such as what I've described above, it's going to be harder to manage stress. Mental stress can cause physical dysfunction and pain, and I've seen stress cause chronic headaches, neck pain, tightness, and overall tension. Chiropractic adjustments bring the body from a sympathetic (fight or flight) state into a parasympathetic state (rest and digest); stress is released, and the body learns a new way of living. The adjustment also gently and powerfully releases stress held in the muscles and tissues of the body, allowing the body to relax and release.

Restorative activities can also help manage stress on a daily basis; it's important to do something, anything, for just *yourself* on a daily basis.

Restorative activities to help manage stress can also look like the following:

- Morning journaling for 15 minutes- ask a question at the top of the page
- Early morning sunrise watching. Research has shown that watching the sunrise may help boost mood, reduce inflammation and depression, and possibly attain better sleep quality at night.
- Stress relieving exercise 10 - 20 minutes a day. Yin Yoga, Pilates, walking, swimming.
- Gratitude exercises for five to ten minutes a day.
- Prayer and daily connection to a Higher Power.
- Meditation (guided or unguided). There are hundreds of these on YouTube or online, as short as a few minutes into longer meditations.
- Anchoring to the present moment and being aware without judgment, just observing yourself in your environment, and being aware of tastes, smells, and sounds will all connect you to the present.
- Intentional times with a dear friend or family member—making time for dinner or coffee *without* children.
- Breathwork via guided videos can shift you out of sympathetic to parasympathetic.
- Grounding: walking barefoot on the Earth and allowing the Earth's gravitational pull to draw you in.
- Rooting: A technique that I've created and found helpful over the years: Sit at the base of a strong tree and imagine connecting the nerve roots of your sacrum to the roots of the tree, allowing the Earth's gravitational pull to draw your energy down. Sit for about 10-15 minutes.
- Epsom salt baths: Not only are these warm baths relaxing, but when dissolved in warm water, Epsom salt is absorbed through the skin and replenishes the level of magnesium in the body. The magnesium helps to produce serotonin, a mood-elevating chemical within the brain that creates a feeling of calm and relaxation.
- Connecting with nature in some fashion for a few minutes a day can help to bring you back to the present moment.

As always, discuss anything with your healthcare providers before implementing it to ensure it is safe and appropriate for your specific needs.

BEING MIND*FUL*

What are your fears about the birthing process? This is a question I always ask my pregnant moms. I'd rather mom be able to discuss what those fears are and find ways to address them either through referrals to a therapist or mindful work.

In the same fashion, what are your fears around child-rearing? What are your worries or concerns? Do you feel you are enough? Do you feel you have enough love to go around?

These are examples of regular thoughts that can often consume us. Having studied the subconscious mind for the last 15 years, I've found that patients often have a pattern they fall into. Since our belief systems are handed down from generation to generation, our grandmothers, and mothers' belief systems around child rearing and what's appropriate or not appropriate can be a big influence in our own minds. At times, if we don't feel we are living up to the way that our elders did things, it can cause stress or anxious feelings within.

As in all things, the first step is to be aware. Are these accurate thoughts? Are they logical? Are we living in a different time than our grandparents or parents? What is true for us and our specific families? Is there a component of trauma? Where does most of your stress come from? Where do your thoughts wander when you're alone? What can we do with the circumstances and what we have been given? Where do we have a sense of control in our lives?

These questions can also be good journaling prompts, where you're writing the question at the top of the notebook and then taking a moment to breathe and free-write whatever comes to your mind out on paper. It's a practice I've been doing for the last 16 years. It's always so good to see what I'm thinking right in front of me on paper and then create (or sit with) possible next steps or next shifts that need to occur in our lives.

Therapy may be an important component of your mental health during the postpartum period. Using therapy or other modalities such as Psych-K, hypnotherapy or other subconscious re-training as needed can be enormously beneficial. Don't suffer in silence! There is absolutely no shame in asking for help or knowing your own limits. Your mental health is extremely important for yourself, your loved ones, and your baby (or babies).

In the Pakistani culture I grew up in, many women have a period of confinement within the house for 40 days after the baby is born in the postpartum period. This is seen as a restorative time after childbirth in which a woman returns to her mother's home, is fed fortifying foods, is exempt from household responsibilities, is taken care of, given massages, pampered, and nourished back to health with healthy foods.

When I was younger, I thought that the 40 days were purely for physical rest, and while that is true, even more important is to replenish the mind from the experience of pregnancy and childbirth. While you may not want to adhere to the 40 days, use the experience of ancient wisdom in your own life. It's a time to take a break and realize that delivering a child could be taxing on the body and mind. Allow others to help you in the first phases of when your new baby has arrived, and *Let Go*! Remember, *done* is better than *perfect*, and it's okay to have others help you so you can heal and focus some of your energy on yourself!

In order for true healing to happen, as a mom, you *must*, even temporarily, place yourself first. It may feel selfish, but it's not; it's actually selfless! This does not mean that your children or the rest of the family are not important; quite the opposite. When your cup is empty, you cannot give to the others in your life, especially your children. You cannot show up 100% for them, your partner/spouse, or any of your loved ones, even the pets.

This is the moment that you will now place your own needs and your own health first so you can restore your health and sense of self. It truly is about making a decision and drawing a line in the sand that *this* is the point where you will make yourself a priority. This decision is an act of self-love and ultimately sends a message to yourself that you are important and worthy of love, attention, and care- first from yourself, then from others.

Many of us get used to pain and discomfort, and it becomes a normal part of our lives. I believe we were meant to thrive, not just survive! We're born to be healthy, vibrant, and well; begin today by transforming your health and living your best life, postpartum and beyond.

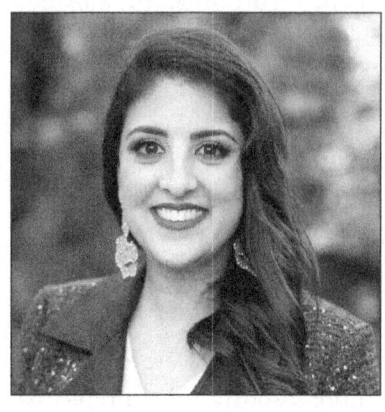

Dr. Irum Tahir is an international speaker, chiropractor, entrepreneur, and business coach. She has worked with organizations in Spanish Harlem, Pakistan, India, Madagascar, and with Syrian refugees to bring chiropractic to thousands of individuals.

Dr. Tahir successfully created High Point Chiropractic Wellness, a family-based wellness practice that has been running independently for the last 17 years. The practice is known as the #1 Pregnancy Chiropractic Center in Upstate New York, has been named best Chiropractic practice four years in a row, and was the recipient of the Excellence in Healthcare award. With multiple doctors and an excellent team, the practice has expanded from Syracuse, New York, to the Washington D.C. area.

A frequent speaker in the chiropractic and medical fields, Dr. Tahir's expertise is in business development, leadership, and practice management. She is an international expert in prenatal and postpartum care and in creating collaboration between MDs, OBs, and chiropractors.

Dr. Tahir has been honored as one of the top 100 Entrepreneurs in the US by the President of the United States. She has been honored at both the White House and the United Nations in the entrepreneurship field, and her popular TED talk on limiting beliefs in the subconscious mind has surpassed a half-million views. Dr. Tahir was named Top 40 Entrepreneurs in New York and Woman of the Year within the chiropractic profession. She has been featured on ABC, in Entrepreneur magazine and the American Chiropractor. She lives in Annapolis, Maryland, with her husband, two boys, and German Shepard, Navy.

Dr. Tahir uses chiropractic, Psych-K, and nutrition to help women heal from within. Find your path to replenish wholeness and live a happy, vibrant life:

To make an appointment, learn about business coaching, or hire Dr. Tahir to speak at your next event, text (315)406-1915

Find her on Instagram: https://www.instagram.com/drirumtahir
https://www.drirumtahir.com
https://www.ignite-spark.com

CHAPTER 18

Embracing Imperfection

REDISCOVERING BODY CONFIDENCE AFTER CHILDBIRTH

Tara De Leon, MS, RSCC, CSCS*D, Author, Speaker, Mama

MY STORY

Ugh, is it already morning? I groan as I awkwardly roll over in bed. *Oooh, gotta pee so bad. Better hurry!* I slowly get up and make my way to the bathroom, not even bothering to put on my glasses.

If I'm lucky, I can get a few more minutes of sleep before my new baby wakes.

The Baby Dude, my nine-day-old son, was sleeping peacefully in his bassinet at the bottom of my bed.

I can't believe he's finally here, I thought as I sat there on the potty. As I finished up and made my way back to my bedroom, my husband started to stir. He opened his eyes as I was walking back through our doorway. "Babe! Don't move!" The urgency in his voice scared me. I couldn't see anything; my body was a hot mess and in no way ready to take on any sort of intruder or whatever. I freeze, silently panicking. "What is it," I ask, terrified.

"There's a spider!"

"Where," I ask.

"Right there!" He replied.

"Where?! What kind of spider?"

"What, I don't know," he tells me, rolling his eyes. Of course, I couldn't see his eyes, but after you've been married seven years, you just know.

At this point, I have no idea how big this spider is or where it is. My postpartum hormones are surging. *It's probably about to descend on my face!*

"Where! Where?" I scream, wringing my hands and squirming around. Mavs wakes up and starts fussing, and I don't even know if this spider is on him or not.

Damn, these stupid eyes! I need to do LASIK.

I'm crying and freaking out, and then I feel some pee on my leg.

I just peed. How is there even anything left in there?

It was then that I felt my milk let down and soak my jammies.

What a look.

Ah, motherhood. The funny thing is I'm not even scared of spiders. Bees or wasps, on the other hand, I would've been out of that room so fast. But spiders, whatever. I just panicked because I didn't know where it was. Isn't it wild that my body peed, cried, and milked all involuntarily? Even after learning so much about the human body, it totally shocked me that this type of reaction was even possible.

How amazing are our bodies? They can grow an entire human in just 40 weeks. Sometimes not even that long. And then, after the baby is born, our bodies can create food for them, most of the time, anyway. We can heal from injuries, grow, and do incredible things with our bodies.

Think for a minute about all the incredible things your body has done. I don't know about you, but my body has run marathons, lifted serious weight, tenderly held tiny animals, grown a baby, made countless meals for those in need, completed triathlons, produced milk for my baby, worked for millions of hours, cried so many tears, birthed my baby, swam with sharks, played tag with kids, walked dogs, hiked mountains, got wicked altitude sickness in those mountains, had passionate sex, held a crying friend, and squeezed my dad's hand as he took his last breath. Does my body look awesome? Not usually. Am I sometimes embarrassed about how my body looks, especially considering what I do for work? Absolutely. It doesn't change the fact that my body is amazing and has done unbelievable things.

On the other hand, your body goes through a ton of changes, none more so than when you conceive, grow, give birth to, and feed a baby. You may not even recognize yourself some days. Did I ever think I would pee, cry, and explode breast milk all over myself all at the same time? Most assuredly, I did not. And like the spider in my room, which, by the way, was the world's smallest spider and was safely on the wall, nowhere near me or my son, it can be scary. These changes are new to us. We may not like them, although I have to admit, my fully engorged boobs, first thing in the morning, were a thing of beauty. It was like a non-surgical boob job for a while anyway. Then once I quit nursing, the image of an orange in a tube sock was a bit more accurate. Everything changes.

Body image is a huge issue I regularly see in postpartum women. I see this in most people, but it's particularly pronounced in postpartum women. Society expects us to bounce back from childbirth as if we didn't just spend the last nine months of our lives growing and changing for this baby. And for some of us, months or even years before that, taking fertility drugs, changing our habits, and praying like never before. Also, the phrases "bounce back" and "get your body back" are 1000% my pet peeves, so you will never hear me talk about doing those things ever. It's not as if we "lost" our bodies and must go find them. Ridiculous. My body and yours do amazing things; let's not forget that. Many mamas come to me talking about their squishy bellies or soft bodies. The reality is that your body went through some serious stuff, and it's going to take time to strengthen it.

The world makes it difficult to cultivate a positive body image by focusing so much on how our bodies look rather than how they perform. My goal is to switch the thought from form to function. Has anyone ever asked you if you've lost all the baby weight yet? Or maybe how much weight you might have gained during pregnancy? It's uncomfortable when people notice your body is changing, even more uncomfortable when they comment on it. When you do experience this, get curious. Why are they observing your body? What do they mean by the comment? Are they just not thinking about how it will affect you, or do they mean harm?

When this happens, I'm giving you permission to walk away from the conversation. Recognizing that it's harmful to you and to others to talk about how bodies look is important. Feel free to remove yourself. This is appropriate even when the conversation is in your own mind about yourself. You have permission to stop that train of thought in its tracks and move on to something else. Life, and especially postpartum life, is hard enough without us beating ourselves up about how we look.

Stacey Sorgen, a Health at Every Size (also known as HAES) aligned adaptive movement coach, offers these alternative suggestions if walking away doesn't work.

1. Ignore it. Change the subject or simply don't answer.
2. Laugh it off in front of others and then approach them later one-on-one.
3. Say, "Please don't comment on my body."
4. Or maybe say, "Maybe you thought I didn't hear you because I was silent or changed the subject, but you hurt me. I would appreciate it if you didn't talk about my body." If they reply with "I'm concerned about your health," hit them with this: "Weight is not an indicator of health. I am happy with who I am. It feels gross to be observed. I am so much more than my body. Have you heard of HAES/Body Neutrality/Body Liberation? I have some book recommendations for you."
5. Be silent and stare for an awkwardly long time. Then ask, "What did you say?" And if they dare repeat themselves, do the silent stare thing again.

Dealing with people's comments about your body can be the hardest part of healing your body image. And yes, body image is something that can be healed. And no, healing your body image doesn't mean changing your body so that it looks like you think it should. Healing your body image is all about healing your mind and recognizing that your value doesn't come from your appearance. Healing body image is a journey that takes time and effort. It starts with confronting your own ideas and core beliefs about bodies. Are all bodies good bodies? Even ones that don't look a certain way? Even ones that don't work the way they're supposed to?

One of the reasons I'm so open about my fertility journey is because it's such a source of shame for so many other women. Many women are devastated and embarrassed that their bodies can't seem to do this one thing. For me, I don't care. I wear contacts, had braces, and color my hair, too. Same, same, same. Not everything works all the time, and that's okay.

It can also be helpful to carefully curate the people around you. Do you have someone in your life that always ends up making you feel bad about yourself? Maybe you limit contact with that person or make sure that when you do see them, you're armed with your self-confidence and a game plan. Check out your social media. Is your entire feed full of diet culture? Go through and start unfollowing people who aren't empowering you to love yourself. Try to find social media accounts that most closely align with your values. That way, when you have a setback, you have a village to fall back on for support, even if it's only through social media.

It's also okay to be sad about not having the body you used to have. Your feelings are valid. We don't want to live in dissatisfaction or even hate forever, so take time to grieve it if you need to. It's totally normal and acceptable to have a sense of grief and loss over your body.

In the movie, "*The Family Man*," Nicholas Cage is psyching himself up to change his first poopy diaper. Pacing back and forth, he says, "You shot the rapids in Kanai. You ran with the bulls in Pamplona. You've jumped out of an airplane over the Mojave Desert, for Christ's sake. You can do this!" While I think it's a little dramatic over changing a diaper, it's a brilliant tool for reminding yourself how badass you are if you might have forgotten.

Allow me to share the story I use to remind myself that I am a fierce warrior goddess.

I went to college at Brigham Young University in Hawaii. I majored in Exercise and Sports Science, which was awesome, by the way. I met many adventurous friends throughout my experience. One day, we took a class field trip to Lanikai to kayak out to the Mokulua Islands. Both islands are seabird sanctuaries protected by the state of Hawaii, but the beach on North Mokulua is open to the public during the day. Located about 30 minutes from campus, I loved going there. The beach was so soft; the sand felt like powdered sugar between my toes. The teal blue water was crystal clear, and the sun was always warm on my skin.

We had so much fun that a few weeks later, a few friends and I decided to go back. It turns out that kayak rentals are expensive, and none of us could afford to rent them. Not wanting to give up on our adventure, we decided to swim out to the islands. Then we would rest for a bit and then swim back.

The islands are a little over a mile offshore, but they looked so close and inviting that none of us thought anything of swimming that far. The water was warm, the afternoon sun was shining, and we were ready! Off we went in pairs. We swam our little hearts out, and I don't know about everyone else, but when we got about halfway out there, I started to second-guess our decision.

Wow, this is harder than I expected.

Once we got past the barrier reef, the waves got some serious size. They weren't huge by Hawaiian standards, but pretty darn big from where I was swimming.

Holy smokes, you're not in the Chesapeake anymore, Tara.

I kept swimming, and eventually, we all made it. Of the six of us, two were fantastic swimmers and didn't appear to be concerned at all. Two were okay-ish, that's where I fit in. I was a lifeguard in college, but we never had to swim that far. And two of us were weak swimmers, and I wasn't sure they'd make it back.

Now, we didn't talk about it and rearrange our groups to put the two strongest swimmers with the two weakest swimmers. That would make too much sense. As we sat there on the beach of the little island, we realized that we actually couldn't rest like we had hoped because the sun was starting to set. We knew that swimming at dusk wasn't recommended due to the increased possibility of a shark attack, so we had to make a choice—spend the night on the island, freezing to death and without any food or water, or get back in right away.

A kayaker beached himself next to us. "Hey, where are your boats?" he asked. "We swam out here," we replied. "Whoa, good for you guys! Better get started back; you don't want to be out here when it gets dark."

With that in mind, we trudged back into the water. I kept my eye on a little pink house on the shore, and, like Dory from Finding Nemo said, "Just keep swimming." I ended up towing my swim buddy back to shore, and as darkness fell, my anxiety heightened. There was no seeing the waves that were coming up behind you. No seeing whatever was swimming beneath you. And no avoiding the rocks and coral that are ubiquitous in that area.

Just keep swimming, just keep swimming. Keep your eye on the pink house and just keep swimming.

Just when I thought my body wouldn't take another stroke, my fingertips hit the sand—the beautiful, powdery, soft sand. I dragged myself up on the beach, grateful to be alive. Two of my friends were already there, and two were still in the water. The funniest part of this story is that we all just got out of the water like, "Whew, glad we made it; where do y'all wanna go eat?" And we went home, showered, and met for dinner an hour later.

The next day we were telling people about our adventure, and we learned that that area is a known tiger shark hangout and not recommended for swimming near the islands. *Ooops.*

It wasn't until much later that I realized how stupid yet completely unbelievable and impressive that was. If I can swim to the Mokulua Islands and back through shark-infested waters at dusk, then I can do anything. My body is awesome. I encourage you to look back through your life at some of the challenging things you've accomplished and pull them out as a beautiful reminder when you're having a bad body image moment.

THE TOOL

HELPFUL MANTRAS FOR BODY IMAGE

Remember, repetition is the key to mantras, so choose one or two that vibe with you and incorporate it into your daily routine. I use the second one, "My body is the least interesting thing about me," as I'm getting dressed in the morning to remind myself that I am fun, fascinating, and fierce.

1. *I am more than my appearance.* Focus on what your body can do rather than what it looks like.
2. *My body is the least interesting thing about me.* You are more than your appearance.
3. *My body deserves love and respect.* You can't hate your body into changing, and it's made a decent home for you since forever, so treat it with respect.
4. *My body is badass, and I am grateful for it.* A gratitude practice is life-changing. Remembering some epic things that you've done with your body can remind you why it's awesome.
5. *I embrace my uniqueness.* Celebrate your individuality and what makes you special.
6. *Self-acceptance, not perfection.* Embrace imperfection; it makes you you!

POSSIBLE TRIGGERS FOR BODY IMAGE

You can't heal your body image by reading one chapter in a book, even a badass chapter in an even more epic book. But you can recognize your body image triggers and learn how to cope with them. Here are just a few that I see frequently.

1. *Trying to squeeze yourself back into clothes that are way too tight.* Every time those clothes rub, chafe, and squeeze you, it will remind you that you are "too big" and could potentially trigger negative body image.
2. *Having people comment on your changing body.* We can't control what other people do or say, but having your response or reaction ready can be helpful. When in doubt, don't hesitate to walk away and take a breath.

3. *Noticing that your body doesn't look like it used to.* I like to Pause and Reframe. Pause, notice the thing, and then reframe it. For example, stretch marks become "badass tiger stripes." Or saggy boobs might become "epic cost-effective baby feeders."
4. *New roles and responsibilities.* Of course you have new roles and responsibilities! You just had a baby, after all! However, adjusting to the new demands of motherhood may shift your focus away from self-care and prioritizing your own body.
5. *Societal Pressures.* Just because people like Kim Kardashian or Becky from down the street returned to their pre-baby body in .7 seconds doesn't mean that they're healthy, have a good body image, or that you need to do anything like they did. For the love of God, please don't do anything like she did. We're all on our own journeys.

Notice your triggers, learn to deal with them, and if you need help healing on your body image journey, go get it. I truly believe the world will be a better place when we have a generation of mamas raising their babies as strong, confident, badass women and setting that example for the generations to come.

PODCAST EPISODES THAT MIGHT BE HELPFUL TO YOU:

Reclaiming Confidence: A Fat Shaming Survival Guide

https://podcasts.apple.com/us/podcast/wellness-rebranded-intuitive-eating-diet-culture-food/id1651744916?i=1000633325423

The Power of Self-Compassion: Unlocking the Path to Wellbeing

https://podcasts.apple.com/us/podcast/wellness-rebranded-intuitive-eating-diet-culture-food/id1651744916?i=1000629317563

Closing Chapter

Hey Hot Mom!

Do you feel a bit more equipped to be healthy, on it, and thriving? My most sincere hope is that you will take the tools from this outstanding compilation of experts and apply them to your lives. Okay, okay, my actual most sincere wish is to never have to do laundry or dishes again, but you hear what I'm saying. The tools we've compiled in this book will absolutely change your life, not only postpartum but throughout your lifespan.

On days you feel like you're barely hanging on, just hang on. There's no award for being that extra Pinterest mom or always having your shizz together. It's okay to just get through it sometimes. Whether we're talking about exercising, meal prepping, body image, mental health, or meditation, the goal of this book is to give you the tools to thrive when you're ready to take that step. If you don't do it all at once, that's just fine. The tools are here when you're ready.

Depending on where you are in your motherhood journey, maybe you're still pregnant (this book makes an awesome baby shower gift, I'm just sayin'!), newly postpartum, or maybe your baby is more of a toddler at this point. It doesn't matter; this book is for you. I've curated a list of some of my favorite, most helpful things for new mamas. I hope you love it and find it useful.

TARA'S FAVORITE THINGS FOR NEW MOMS

1. A plan to divide and conquer. If you have a spouse or partner, determine who will research what. Safe sleep, car seats, strollers, feeding, swaddling, discipline, dealing with crazy in-laws, put it all on the list. As mothers, we tend to take on more than our fair share of the mental load. Decide together which parts you will each be responsible for and stick to it.

2. A progressive relaxation technique that will help you calm down, fall asleep, or even reset yourself after a stressful situation. Maybe a public meltdown? I recorded this as an episode on my podcast, Wellness Rebranded, and you can do it in 30 seconds or an hour. It's made to fit into your life as you need it. Check it out here: https://podcasts.apple.com/us/podcast/wellness-rebranded-intuitive-eating-diet-culture-food/id1651744916

3. One of my amazing co-authors, Elizabeth Harris, teaches a class on Raising Intuitive Eaters. I really believe that if we as mothers can change the way we look at food and behave around food, our kids and generations to come will be in a much healthier place. I took her class, and it completely changed the way I feed my child. https://elizabethharrisnutrition.com/course You can also listen to a podcast we did on that topic here: https://podcasts.apple.com/us/podcast/wellness-rebranded-intuitive-eating-diet-culture-food/id1651744916

4. Making sure my baby was sleeping safely is a HUGE priority for me. When I was pregnant with my son, I dug deep into safe sleep and found this incredible Facebook group that, most importantly, uses evidence-based recommendations only. The tone of the group can be a bit brusque, but it's only because they have your baby's safety at heart, and they aren't going to sugarcoat anything to save your feelings. You can find it here: https://www.facebook.com/groups/399370380437680

5. My all-time favorite baby purchase: The Doona Car Seat Stroller. This thing made my life so much easier for that first year. I loved it so much that I still wish they somehow made one big enough to fit my three-and-a-half-year-old.

6. My other favorite baby purchase: a Keekaroo Diaper Changing Pad. Oh, baby had a blowout all over it? No worries, just wipe it off and continue your life. No extra laundry to do, especially with baby poop on it.

7. My favorite feeding tool was the Kiinde system. It is a system of milk storage bags that you can pump into and then pop a nipple onto it and feed directly from it. No more dirty bottles, ever. Just wash the nipple and go! I liked it so much (anything that eliminates dishes is a big win in my book) that I even mixed up formula in them after my breastfeeding journey had ended.

8. A lactation consultant if you are planning on breastfeeding. It seems so simple, right? Put baby on boob, let 'em eat, then burp them, and you're done, right? Not quite. I'd preemptively book a session with one in the first few days of being home.

9. It's not really a thing, but it's still worth mentioning. Your relationship with your spouse will change. He's probably as new to this as you are. He also might feel a bit helpless, alone, left out, whatever because you have done most of the work so far. He still needs you. You still need him. Don't stop dating him just because your family is bigger. You need each other, so don't go acting like you don't. Plus, dating is fun, especially when you already know that your date isn't a creeper. Or maybe you know he is, but you're obviously into that. In the beginning, it can feel daunting to fit in a date night, but make it a regular thing, and it'll help you still feel like you, and y'all still feel like y'all. Even free dates are good! My hubby and I used to get a babysitter and just go drive around for a little while.

10. Take time for yourself. I know this is hard. We are programmed to think that it's all about the baby, and we should put ourselves last. No. You can't pour from an empty cup. You need to put your oxygen mask on before you help others with theirs. Figure this out so that you can still be you and not always mom, wife, maid, chef, daughter, sister, and all the other hats we wear. You still need to be you. By doing so, everyone else will get the best version of you, too.

11. Secondary infertility is a thing, and it's super common. Don't mess around with this; if something doesn't seem right, go see your doctor or just go straight to Shady Grove Fertility or another fertility specialist. I wouldn't be a mama without them, this book wouldn't exist, and my whole life would be crazy different.

12. Mom's Special Healing Spray. You probably won't need this until you have a toddler, but it's essential. When I was pregnant, I asked my mom the actual name of her special healing spray that she always used on us. It was in a little white spray bottle with a red cross and an aloe vera leaf on it. I wanted to make sure I had some on hand for when we needed it. Guess what she told me? It was freaking water in a spray bottle. But because she told us it would make us feel better, we believed her, embarrassingly, until I was like 36 years old. But it got us through some tough injuries as kids, so definitely keep this on hand. I couldn't find a bottle that looked legit, so I got a Band-Aid antibacterial spray bottle and used that.

13. Therapy. As a society, we don't do a great job of taking care of our postpartum mamas. We get that six-week postpartum checkup where they ask how the baby is, if we feel okay, and then tell our husbands we're open for business again. That's pretty much it. I'm sure I don't have to tell you; we need more than that. We deserve more than that. Find an amazing therapist and go check in as needed.

14. The book called "There Are Way Worse Moms Than You" by Glenn Boozan. We all have our days where the momming ain't momming and you feel like trash about yourself, your parenting, and probably everything else. This book is a super short, quick, easy read about moms in the animal kingdom who we probably wouldn't consider to be the best parents. For example, if a panda has twins, she abandons one because she's not about that twin life. Koala mamas will feed her babies her own poop. These and other true facts from the animal kingdom offer a hilarious reality check on what constitutes "good parenting" so that we human moms can relax and realize that we got this.

15. The Village. Ah, yes, the elusive village that is supposed to be all around us. Where is it, right? I'm convinced that many of us don't have a village, have a tiny village, or must pay for our village. You know what? Take that village however you can get it. Outsource what you can. Have a cleaning service come in to help with cleaning and laundry. Maybe you do one of those meal prep services. Have a couple of babysitters that you can call in an emergency. You can do it on your own, but it completely sucks to do it like that. Organize as much as you can to take things off your plate before it becomes an emergency. What happens in an emergency? Make those plans now. Also, recognize that your village might change over time. You might outgrow people, or people might drift out of the village. That's okay. Your needs will change, too. Look for people who you can offer support to their village as well. The village is supposed to benefit everyone.

So, there you go, Hot Mom, a few tools to add to your new mom toolkit. Go out there and remember who you are. Empowered women empower women, so don't forget to share the hot mom tools with others. You got this!

Acknowledgments

This book would have never happened without the support of so many people. First on the list is my amazing husband, Marcus De Leon. From wrangling the Baby Dude so I could write to being a sounding board for my ideas, you've always been there, helping and supporting me along the way. I love you!

Next would be my own mama and my little bro, Chris. Thanks for being a fantastic cheering squad and support system. To my dad, even though you passed on in 2014, I felt your presence while writing this book and more importantly continue to feel it guiding me while parenting Maverick. I know that you're so proud of me and not at all surprised that I'm doing cool things. Miss you so much.

To Laura and her amazing team at Brave Healer Productions, thank you all for making my dream, this book, a reality. Holding my hand and walking me through the process of publishing a book, step by step, is exactly what I needed. I still can't believe we did it!

To my business coach, AliceAnne Loftus. Girl, thanks for forcing me out of my comfort zone and planting this seed. I needed the push and I have enjoyed the journey. I'm so glad you're in my life.

And lastly, to all my friends and clients who have endured my endless chatter about this project for the past few months, who have read the early drafts and given me valuable feedback, edits, critiques, and encouragement, thank you. Your support means more than you probably even realize. Thanks for putting up with me.

It's been said that to the world, you are a mother, but to your family, you are the world. Just because you are the world, doesn't mean you don't deserve to be healthy, on it, and thriving. It means you have a responsibility to be so.

~ Tara De Leon

Made in the USA
Middletown, DE
17 April 2024